Pharmacology for technicians
Workbook

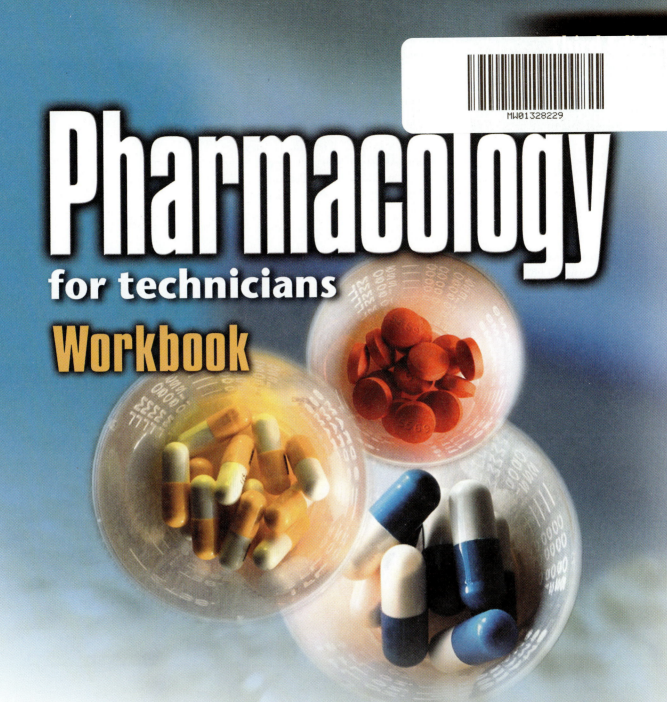

Don A. Ballington, MS
Midlands Technical College
Columbia, South Carolina

Mary M. Laughlin, PharmD, MEd
Regional Medical Center
Memphis, Tennessee

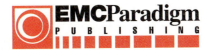

Senior Editor Christine Hurney
Editorial Assistant Susan Capecchi
Copyeditor Judy Peacock
Cover and Text Designer Leslie Anderson

Publishing Management Team
George Provol, Publisher; Janice Johnson, Vice President of Marketing; Jeanne Allison, Acquisitions Editor; Shelley Clubb, Electronic Design and Production Manager

ISBN 0-7638-2213-2
Product Number 03655

Care has been taken to verify the accuracy of information presented in this book. The authors, editors, and publisher, however, cannot accept responsibility for errors or omissions or for consequences from application of the information in this book and make no warranty, expressed or implied, with respect to its content.

Some of the product names used in this book have been used for identification purposes only and may be trademarks or registered trademarks of their respective manufacturers.

© 2006, 2003, 1999 by Paradigm Publishing Inc.
    Published by **EMC**Paradigm
    875 Montreal Way
    St. Paul, MN 55102
    (800) 535-6865
    E-mail: educate@emcp.com
    Website: www.emcp.com

All rights reserved. Permission is granted by the publisher to reproduce portions of this guide for educational use at a single location.

Printed in the United States of America.

10 9 8 7 6 5 4 3

Contents

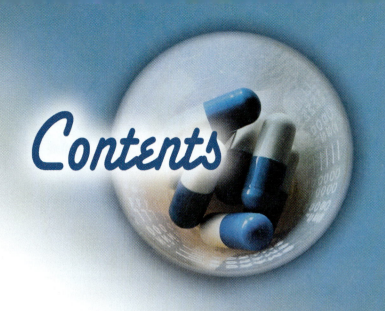

Preface .... *iv*

UNIT 1 Introduction to Pharmacology 1
Chapter 1 The Evolution of Medicinal Drugs 3
Chapter 2 Basic Concepts of Pharmacology 9
Chapter 3 Dispensing of Pharmacologic Agents 15

UNIT 2 Anti-Infectives 19
Chapter 4 Antibiotics 21
Chapter 5 Therapy for Fungi and Viruses 31

UNIT 3 Narcotic Pain Relievers, Neurologicals, and Psychiatric Drugs 43
Chapter 6 Anesthetics, Analgesics, and Narcotics 45
Chapter 7 Antidepresseants, Antipsychotics, Antianxiety Agents, and Alcoholism ... 53
Chapter 8 Anticonvulsants and Drugs to Treat Other CNS Disorders 63

UNIT 4 Respiratory, GI, Renal, and Cardiac Drugs 71
Chapter 9 Respiratory Drugs 73
Chapter 10 Gastrointestinal Drugs and Related Diseases 85
Chapter 11 Urinary System Drugs 95
Chapter 12 Cardiovascular Drugs 105

UNIT 5 Muscle Relaxants, Nonnarcotic Analgesics, Hormones, and Topicals 115
Chapter 13 Muscle Relaxants, Nonnarcotic Analgesics, and Anti-Inflammatories ... 117
Chapter 14 Hormones 127
Chapter 15 Topicals, Ophthalmics, and Otics 137

UNIT 6 Chemotherapy and Nutritional and Alternative Substances .. 147
Chapter 16 Recombinant Drugs and Chemotherapy 149
Chapter 17 Vitamins, Nutritional and Alternative Supplements, Antidotes, and Emergencies 159

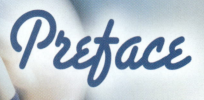

Preface

This workbook has been prepared to accompany the text *Pharmacology for Technicians, Third Edition* by Don Ballington and Mary M. Laughlin. Along with the textbook, Encore CD, and supporting Internet Resource Center, this workbook is designed to help students develop a commitment to the pharmacy field with the hope that, as pharmacy technicians, they will be challenged by this constantly changing field and motivated to learn more about the body and the drugs that heal and improve the lives of patients.

This workbook provides exercises for each chapter of the textbook. Instructors may choose to assign these exercises as a take home test or homework assignments. These exercises can also be used to support independent study of the textbook content. Some exercises may require students to do drug-specific research, using resources other than the textbook.

Workbook exercises for chapters in Unit 1 focus on the important foundation material presented in that unit, specifically the science of pharmacology and the study of pharmacokinetics. Drug-specific exercises do not start until Unit 2.

The following exercises are provided for chapters in Units 2–6.

- Reading Drug Labels and Medication Orders requires students to apply literacy skills and drug-dispensing knowledge.
- Understanding the Larger Medical Context asks students to focus on medical issues such as disease states, anatomy and physiology, and drug classes in order to demonstrate an understanding of why certain drugs are prescribed, how they are used, and their pharmacokinetic effects.
- Communicating in the Pharmacy helps students develop skills communicating to patients and other health care professionals about pharmacy-related issues. In addition, these exercises help technicians understand what type of information a technician can communicate to a patient and what type of information should be communicated by the pharmacist.
- Dispensing and Storing Drugs asks students to identify storage requirements and auxiliary labels necessary to ensure patient safety and compliance.
- Putting Safety First expands on the text's focus on safety by asking students to compare presented doses with standard or typical doses in order to recognize potential errors as well as to identify potential drug interactions.
- Puzzling the Technician and Puzzling Terminology crossword puzzles are a fun way to reinforce chapter concepts and terminology.

Additional instructional support is provided on the Encore CD included with each textbook. For the chapters in Units 2 through 6, the Encore CD includes Drug Drills and Fast Drug Facts based on the drug tables presented in the text. Drug Drills include matching exercises designed to reinforce the learning of brand and generic drug names, drug classes, and drug uses. The Fast Drug Facts further reinforce the learning of drug names and drug classes and also include audio pronunciations of all of the generic drug names.

The Encore CD also includes interactive review questions that students can use to test their knowledge of concepts presented in the book. There are two levels of tests—book and chapter—and each level functions in two different modes. In the Review mode, the student receives immediate feedback on each test item and a report of his or her total score. In the reportable Practice Test mode, the results are e-mailed to both the student and the instructor. The Encore CD also includes a complete glossary and image bank created from key illustrations from the textbook.

The Internet Resource Center for this title at www.emcp.com provides additional chapter study resources including PowerPoint slide shows, interactive drug name flash cards, flash cards containing drug facts from the chapter drug tables in .rtf format, lecture and study notes, as well as additional crossword puzzles. These resources can be downloaded and adapted to meet each student's particular study needs.

The authors would like to thank the editorial team at Paradigm Publishing, Inc. as well as the following contributors for their involvement in developing this workbook.

David Mangan, PharmD
Boston Medical Center
Boston, Massachusetts

Scott Shepard, PharmD, RPh
Boston, Massachusetts

Mary Ann Stuhan, RPh
Cuyahoga Community College
Cleveland, Ohio

The authors and editorial staff encourage your feedback on the text and its supplements. Please reach us by clicking the "Contact Us" button at www.emcp.com.

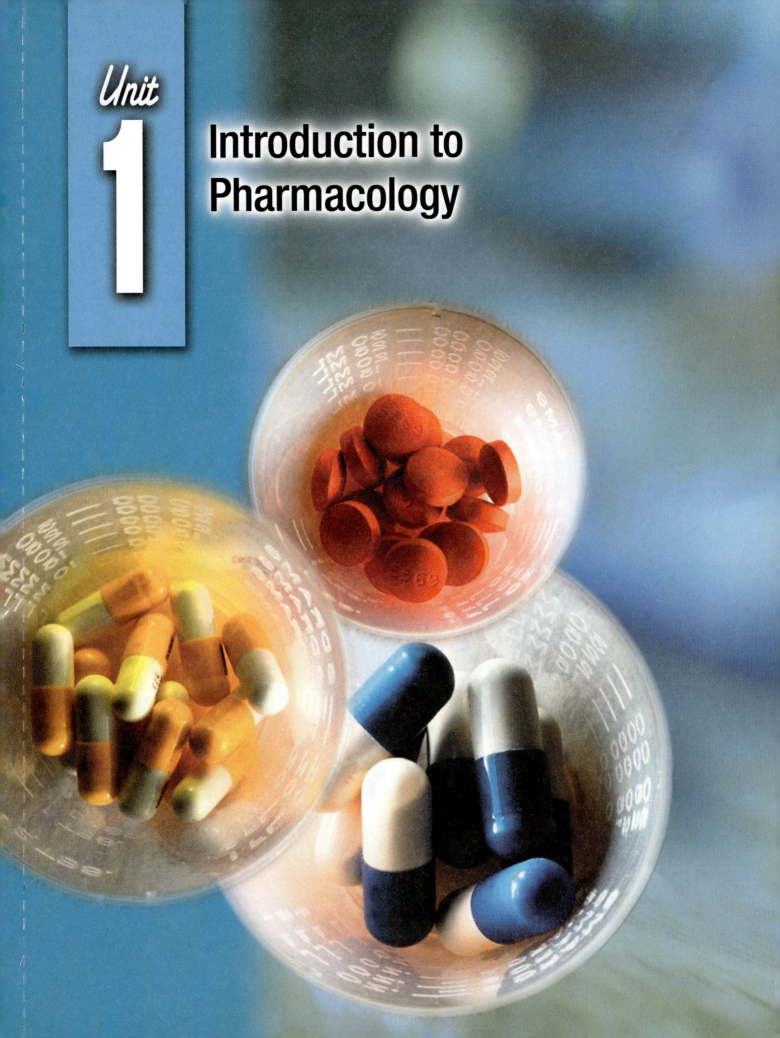

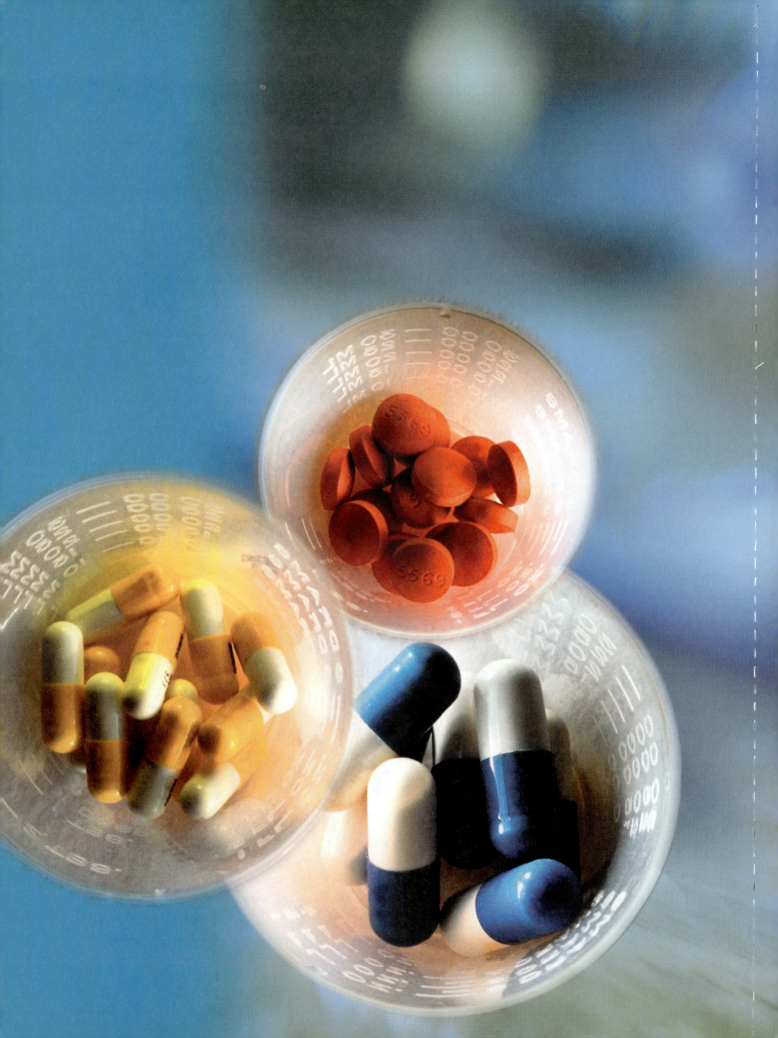

The Evolution of Medicinal Drugs

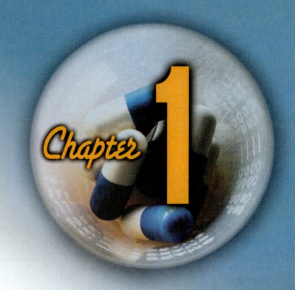

UNDERSTANDING PHARMACOLOGY AND PHARMACOKINETICS

1. A company is trying to market a new antiseptic solution that prevents the spread of disease on hands and surgical equipment. The marketing department wants a catchy name for the product, based on the name of a pioneer in the field of chemical sterilization. What two individuals would you choose, and how are they important?.

   _____
   _____

2. You are applying for a pharmacy technician job at a retail pharmacy in another state. When you read the job description, you notice the following tasks:

   a. transferring prescriptions
   b. demonstrating to asthmatics how to use a metered dose inhaler
   c. preparing prescription labels
   d. maintaining allergy information in the pharmacy system
   e. counseling diabetics with regard to insulin needle use

   Which of these requirements should not be part of the job description?

   _____
   _____

3. How can a patient obtain a schedule I drug?

   _____

4. Why are the achievements of Claude Bernard important to the science of pharmacology?

   _____
   _____

Name _____ Date _____

5. Put these groups related to pharmaceutical practice in order according to the year of their creation. Start with the earliest formed.

   APhA   USP

   FDA   DEA

   _____

6. You are reading a newspaper ad about a drug named BPPA469 for the treatment of osteoarthritis. The ad is recruiting healthy adults, ages 18 to 45 years, to take the drug and to come in once a week to be examined while on BPPA469. What phase of a clinical trial do you think BPPA469 is in? Explain your answer.

   _____

7. A pharmaceutical company is attempting to market a product with the brand name Rivernex and the generic name superatenolol. The drug is a modified form of atenolol that has a lower incidence of hypotension. What is unacceptable about the company's generic naming of the drug?

   _____

8. If you were a student of Galen, what would you consider the sources of disease to be?

   _____
   _____

9. Two drugs come on the market for the treatment of sickle cell disease. One of the sources is a synthetically derived oral tablet, and the other is a recombinant subcutaneous injection. Both are given daily. Which would you assume to have a lower cost? Why?

   _____

10. Would a vaccine be considered a therapeutic or a prophylactic drug? Explain.

    _____
    _____

Fill in the blanks.

11. During phase II of a clinical trial, patients are randomized to take either an active drug or a(n) _____.

12. Methotrexate should never be used by pregnant women because of demonstrated harm to the fetus. That would put the drug in FDA Pregnancy Category _____.

13. A good place to look to see if a generic drug is interchangeable with a brand-name drug would be the _____.

14. To be made available without a prescription, a legend drug must have its status changed to _____.

15. Pharmacy technicians must be recertified every _____ years by the PTCB.

16. The use of _____ drugs help to keep the overall cost of healthcare down.

17. After the patent expires on the drug Trailhex (aeronitriptan), the generic product will be known as _____.

18. Valerius Cordis published the _____ in 1546.

19. The *Pharmacopoeia of the United States* was published by the _____.

20. Metoprolol tartrate and metoprolol succinate are examples of the same chemical available as two different _____.

21. Homeopathic remedies use _____ doses of drugs.

22. Each drug seeking marketing status in the United States must have submitted and received an approved _____.

23. Title II of the Comprehensive Drug Abuse prevention and Control Act of 1970 designated five schedules for _____ according to drugs' probability of abuse.

24. Insulin was first isolated by _____.

25. In a(n) _____ study, neither trail participants nor research staff knows which subjects are in the experimental group and which are part of the control group.

PUZZLING THE TECHNICIAN

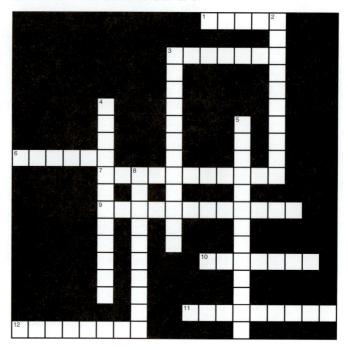

Across

1. drug name that can only be used by the company that developed the drug
3. inactive substance without any known pharmacological activity
6. sole right to manufacture a new drug
7. first to dissect the human body
9. chemical beneficial for sterilizing equipment
10. discovered penicillin in 1945
11. first antibiotic
12. wrote *The Book of Life*

Down

2. wrote *de Materia Medica*
3. study of drugs and their interactions with the systems of living animals
4. synonym for early pharmacists
5. when phase IV clinical trials occur
8. first to use the concept of individual drugs instead of potions

PUZZLING TERMINOLOGY

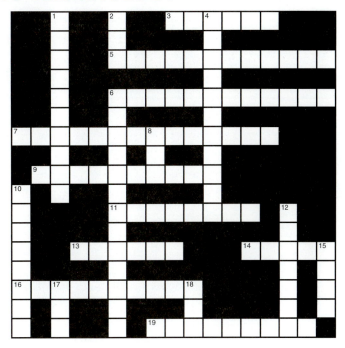

Across

3. a government grant that gives a drug company the sole right to manufacture a drug for a certain number of years
5. early pharmacists and/or their shops
6. the science of drugs and their interactions with the systems of living animals
7. official listings of medicinal preparations
9. one licensed to prepare and sell or dispense drugs and compounds and to fill prescriptions
11. the name that describes a drug's molecular makeup
13. a drug sold only by prescription and labeled "Rx only"
14. the name under which the manufacturer markets a drug; also known as the trade name
16. a drug with potential for abuse is called this type of substance
19. Greek word meaning a magic spell, remedy, or poison

Down

1. therapeutics in which diseases are treated by administering minute doses of drugs capable of producing in healthy patients symptoms like those of the disease being treated
2. the agency of the federal government responsible for ensuring the safety of drugs and food prepared for the market
4. drugs that relieve symptoms of a disease
6. the study and identification of natural sources of drugs
8. a drug sold without a prescription
10. trials in which drugs are tested on humans; used to determine drug safety and efficacy
12. an inactive substance with no treatment value
15. a medicinal substance used to change the way a living organism functions; also called a medication
17. request for FDA approval of a new pharmaceutical for sale and marketing in the United States
18. the branch of the U.S. Justice Department responsible for regulating sale and use of drugs

Basic Concepts of Pharmacology

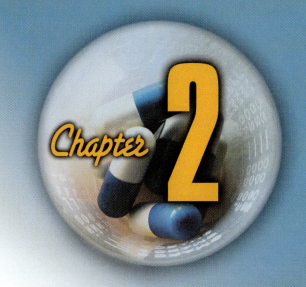

Chapter 2

UNDERSTANDING PHARMACOLOGY AND PHARMACOKINETICS

1. Heart rate increases when beta-1 receptors are stimulated. A patient takes a drug which, binds on the beta receptors, and experiences an increase in heart rate. Was the drug a beta antagonist or a beta agonist? Explain why.

2. Stimulation of beta-2 receptors in the lungs help to open airways during breathing. The patient in question 1 also experiences less bronchoconstriction when taking the drug. What does that tell you about the selectivity of that drug?

3. Which will have a faster onset of action, metoprolol 5 mg intravenous push or metoprolol 50 mg by mouth? Why?

4. Ciclopirox (Penlac) is an antifungal used to treat onychomycosis, a type of nail fungus. The directions say to apply the lacquer to each nail daily. Will the ciclopirox have a local or system effect? Why?

5. For many cases of infective endocarditis, the combination of gentamicin and ampicillin has been shown to be more effective than using each drug individually. The combination also allows the patient to avoid toxicities associated with the higher doses of gentamicin needed for separate dosing. How would you categorize the relationship of gentamicin and ampicillin when used together?

6. Rifampin is a CYP450 3A4 inducer. If a patient is on other drugs that are metabolized by the same isoenzymes, what would you expect to happen to the levels of those drugs when taken in conjunction with rifampin?

7. Mrs. Holly, a cancer patient, has been on high doses of Oxycontin for six months for pain. Her medication is being managed by an oncologist. Mrs. Holly does not experience euphoria when taking the prescribed dosage. Is she dependent on or addicted to the Oxycontin? Explain.

8. Nitroglycerin has been shown to be less pharmacologically active when administered for more than 24 consecutive hours. What could this be attributed to?

9. You read in a medical journal about a patient who developed an enlarged liver after taking a drug that has been available for 15 years. Although the enlarged liver can definitely be attributed to the drug, no such reaction has previously been reported. Is the response in this case allergic, anaphylactic, or idiosyncratic?

10. Two drugs are both anticholinergics. To have equal effects, drug A has to be dosed six times a day and drug B has to be dosed two times a day. Which drug has the longer duration of action? Explain your answer.

11. Phenytoin has a plasma protein binding of about 90% that is exclusively attributed to albumin. If a patient has a total phenytoin level of 15 mcg/mL, and has normal albumin, what would be the expected free phenytoin level?

Fill in the blanks.

12. The _____ prevents many drugs from penetrating the brain.

13. Vancomycin is usually dosed every 12 hours. If a dose was administered at 10:00 a.m., and the concentration of the drug in the blood had fallen to its lowest level at 9:30 p.m., that level would be considered a _____.

14. General anesthetics are excreted by the kidney, liver, and respiratory system. The sum excretion of all these systems is known as total body _____.

15. Many geriatric patients experience a condition called gastroparesis, which greatly delays gastric emptying time. You would expect this condition would also delay drug _____.

16. Patients with impaired liver function who take drugs that are not renally excreted might expect drugs to be present for a _____ amount of time in the blood compared to patients with normal liver function.

17. Drugs that extensively undergo first-pass effect will have a lower _____ than those that do not.

18. Digoxin levels should be between 0.8 ng/mL and 2 ng/mL. A reading between those two numbers is considered to be in the _____.

19. A drug has a blood plasma concentration of 20 mcg/mL. Ten hours later, the plasma concentration is 5 mcg/mL. This drug has a half-life of _____ hours.

20. Patients with a history of uncontrolled hypertension should not receive any type of decongestants. Uncontrolled hypertension is an example of a _____ for decongestants.

21. In order for a drug to be absorbed by the GI tract, it must be _____.

22. The two major routes for excretion are the liver and the _____.

23. _____ bind to a receptor site and block the action of the endogenous messenger or other drugs.

24. The overall pharmacokinetic process is known by the acronym _____.

25. Drug A is a mu-receptor agonist; drug B is a mu-receptor antagonist. When given together, the actions of drug B predominate. Drug B has a greater _____ for the mu receptor.

26. In combination, cilastatin prevents imipenem from being renally eliminated. Cilastatin itself is not pharmacologically active against bacteria. Cilastatin _____ the effect of imipenem.

PUZZLING THE TECHNICIAN

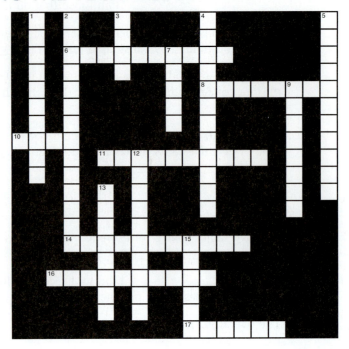

Across

6. M in ADME
8. estrogen agonists will only work on cells with an estrogen _____
10. number of half-lives for a drug to be considered essentially completely eliminated from the body
11. A in ADME
14. E in ADME
16. process that slows or blocks enzyme activity
17. type of alternative medicine

Down

1. action of one drug negates the action of a second drug
2. what an allergic reaction is based on
3. upper limit of a drug's concentration in the blood
4. D in ADME
5. when two drugs alter the efficacy or blood levels of one another
7. disease of this organ decreases overall protein binding
9. an effect expected from excess dosing
12. a drug's ability to dissolve in body fluids
13. combined effect of two drugs, equal to the sum of the effects of each drug taken alone
15. lowest level of a drug in the blood

PUZZLING TERMINOLOGY

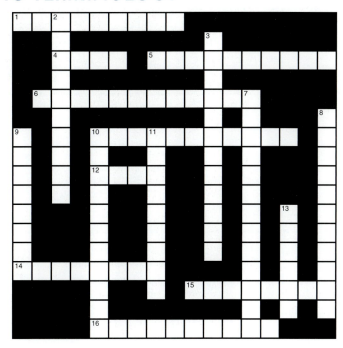

Across

1. dependence characterized by perceived need to take a drug to attain its psychological and physical effects
4. the top or upper limit of a drug's concentration in the blood
5. the process whereby a drug blocks enzyme activity and impairs the metabolism of another drug
6. in this type of response there is immediate life-threatening respiratory distress, usually followed by vascular collapse and shock
10. the property of a receptor site that enables it to bind only with a particular chemical messenger
12. the quantity of a drug administered at one time
14. this type of effect or action of a drug has a generalized, all-inclusive effect on the body
15. in this type of response the immune system overreacts to an otherwise harmless substance
16. a drug's ability to dissolve in body fluids

Down

2. state in which a person's body has adapted physiologically and psychologically to a drug and cannot function without it
3. process by which a drug moves from the blood into other body fluids and tissues to its sites of action
7. point at which no clinical response occurs with increased dosage
8. an action of a drug that is confined to a specific part of the body
9. drugs that bind to a particular receptor site and trigger the cell's response in a manner similar to the action of the body's own chemical messenger
10. secondary responses to a drug other than the primary therapeutic effect for which the drug was intended
11. rate at which a drug is eliminated from a specific volume of blood per unit of time
13. the lowest level of a drug in the blood

Name Date

Dispensing of Pharmacologic Agents

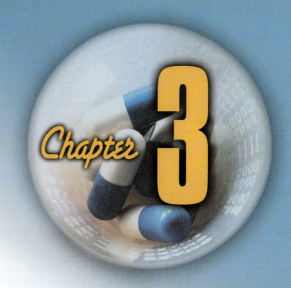

Chapter 3

UNDERSTANDING PHARMACOLOGY AND PHARMACOKINETICS

1. How is it possible for a patient to achieve relief with sublingual nitroglycerin when you know that usually the oral route has an absorption phase of 15 to 30 minutes?

2. What is the route of choice for general anesthetics and why?

3. If a patient is vomiting and IV antiemetics are not available, what other route could be considered?

4. What are two reasons why patients with physical disabilities sometimes have difficulty using inhaled medications?

5. Why might Zantac need to be dose-adjusted in the elderly? (Hint: 30% to 70% of a Zantac dose is excreted unchanged in the urine.)

6. How many different vaccinations should a child have received by the age of six months?

7. Breastfed newborns begin developing their immunity through the antibodies contained in breast milk. Is this active or passive immunity?

8. Some children are genetically predisposed to autoimmune hepatitis. What would be the best strategy to treat this disease?

Name _____ Date _____

9. A pediatric patient, admitted to the emergency room because of an asthma attack, has required corticosteroids to control the inflammation. What type of vaccine should be avoided in this type of patient?

_____

10. How is it possible for a patient to have positive tuberculin skin tests and still have no signs or symptoms of active disease?

_____

Fill in the blanks.

11. The only vaccination on the pediatric schedule that does not require a booster is _____.

12. The _____ is the part of a prescription that tells the patient how to take the medication.

13. Using MSO$_4$ as an abbreviation for morphine sulfate is dangerous because it can easily be confused with _____.

14. The _____ route bypasses the first-pass effect and increases bioavailability.

15. The _____ route uses skin absorption as a mode of delivery for medication.

16. Elderly patients generally have decreased exercise _____ because of age-related degeneration of the cardiovascular system.

17. The decrease in testosterone production experienced by elderly men is an example of _____.

18. Having too many medications to take can cause a decrease in patient _____.

19. Synthetic vaccines contain _____ that cause the body to form an immune response to a certain disease.

20. Histamine is produced in the _____.

21. Nizatidine (Axid) is an example of an _____ blocker.

22. A histamine reaction causes _____ of blood vessels.

23. _____ labels remind patients how to take their medication.

PUZZLING THE TECHNICIAN

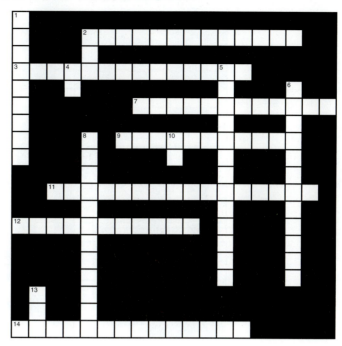

Across

2. endogenous compound that causes uterine and smooth muscle contraction
3. type of protein system that mediates an allergic reaction
7. SC
9. H_1 receptors are populated in this system
11. H_2 receptors are populated in this system
12. ac
14. oral, IM, rectal, and transdermal are all routes of _____

Down

1. hives
2. as needed
4. as directed
5. IM
6. term for having a multiple-drug regimen to treat disease states
8. an order for a medication written by a practitioner to be filled by a pharmacist
10. by mouth
13. four times a day

PUZZLING TERMINOLOGY

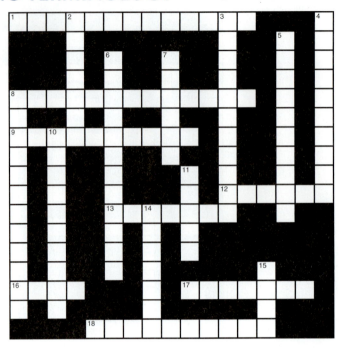

Across

1. not related to disease
8. administration of a medication by injecting it into a muscle; abbreviated IM
9. administration of a drug by placing a tablet under the tongue
12. immunity against disease that occurs as a result of coming into contact with an infectious agent or an inactivated part of such an agent administered by a vaccine
13. medication applied to the surface of the skin or mucous membranes
16. administration of a medication through the ear
17. a state of heightened sensitivity as a result of exposure to a particular substance
18. administration of medication by injection not by way of the alimentary canal

Down

2. administration of a medication by mouth in either solid form or in liquid form
3. administration of a medication through the skin
4. a patient's adherence to the dose schedule and other requirements of the specified regimen
5. administration of a medication through the eye
6. process by which the immune system is stimulated to acquire protection against a specific disease; usually achieved by use of a vaccine
7. administration of a drug by placing a tablet between the cheek and gums
8. administration of a medication drop by drop
10. an endogenous chemical that causes contraction of intestinal, uterine, and bronchial smooth muscle
11. this type of infection is restricted to or pertains to one area of the body
14. immunity against disease as the result of receiving antibodies that were formed by another person or animal who developed them in response to being infected with the disease
15. another term for peroral

Unit 2

Anti-Infectives

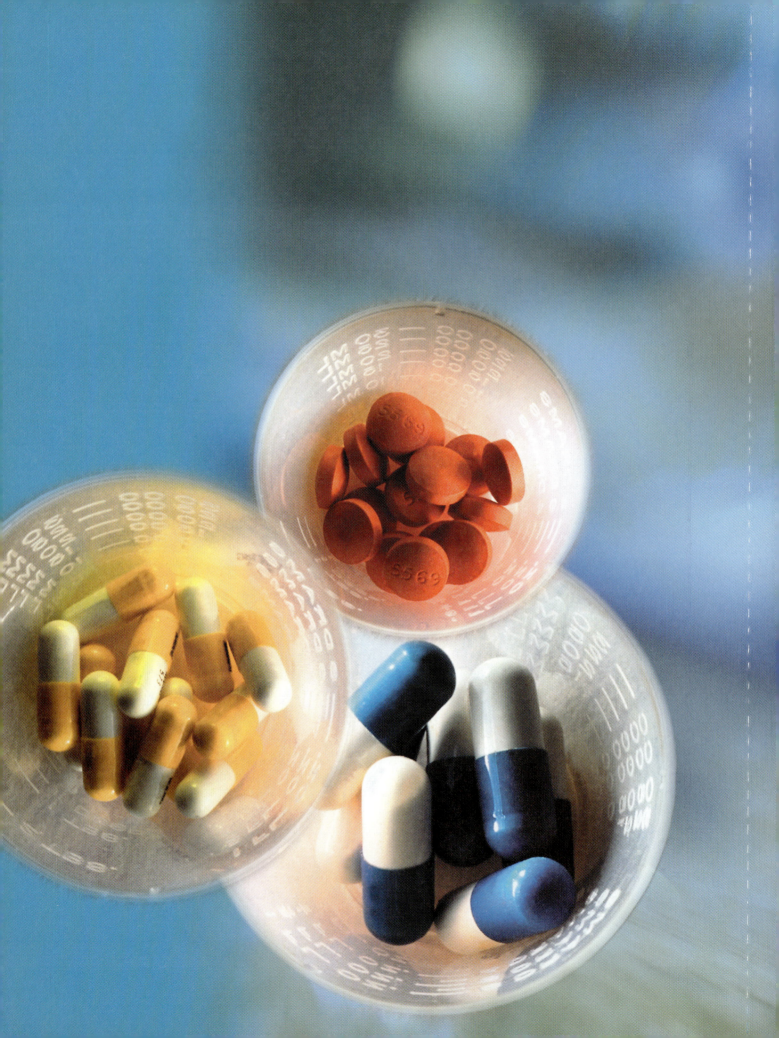

Antibiotics

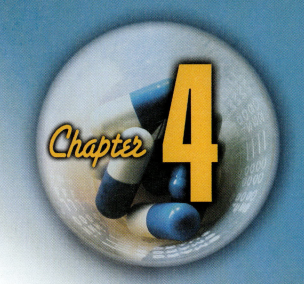

Chapter 4

READING DRUG LABELS AND MEDICATION ORDERS

1. A patient brings in the following prescription, and the drug label shown is the product available in the pharmacy.

    Amoxil 250 mg/5 mL suspension; take 1 tsp tid x 7 days

   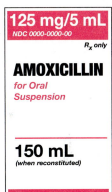

   125 mg/5 mL
   NDC 0000-0000-00
   Rx only
   AMOXICILLIN
   for Oral Suspension
   150 mL
   (when reconstituted)

   a. Since the concentration requested in the prescription is not available, what would the dosing instructions be for the available product? Provide the answer using both teaspoonsful and milliliters. (*Note:* 1 tsp = 5 mL. This and other equivalencies are available in the Pharmacy Library section of this book's Internet Resource Center (IRC) at www.emcp.com.)

   _____
   _____

   b. Using the drug shown in the label, how many milliliters would you dispense to meet the dosing requirements for the entire treatment period? (Do not assume any wasted medication.)

   _____

   c. How many milligrams are prescribed for the patient to take in one day?

   _____

2. A 1 g dose of ceftriaxone is to be administered intramuscularly. The physician states that the patient is an elderly woman who does not have venous access. The following label shows the drug to be administered.

   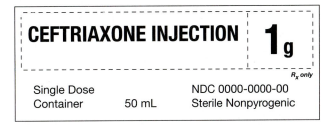

   CEFTRIAXONE INJECTION **1 g**
   Rx only
   Single Dose Container   50 mL   NDC 0000-0000-00   Sterile Nonpyrogenic

Name _____   Date _____

a. How will you reconstitute the vial, and what will the resulting concentration be?

b. What will be the required volume for this dose?

3. You receive the following prescription.

℞ Bactrim DS; 1 tab PO bid x 3d

a. What directions should be on the dispensed prescription label?

b. How many tablets will be dispensed for the duration of therapy?

4. You receive an order in your IV room that is for gentamicin 400 mg. How many milliliters of the following gentamicin would you use to make the dose?

NDC 0000-0000-00
GENTAMICIN
Injection, USP equivalent to
40 mg/mL
20 mL multiple dose vial
For IM or IV use.
R_x only

5. Mr. Duncan is starting on vancomycin 1.5 g IV q12h. The maximum concentrations for direct infusion are 5 mg/mL for peripheral and 10 mg/mL for central. Use the common solution bag sizes (50 mL, 100 mL, 150 mL, 250 mL, 500 mL, 1000 mL) to determine the final volume.

a. What solution would be used for peripheral infusion, and which solution bag would be used?

b. What would be the solution for central infusion, and which solution bag would be used?

6. Your hospital pharmacy makes a fortified tobramycin eyedrop that is 13.6% in a 10 mL bottle. How many milligrams are in the bottle of eyedrops?

7. You have an unusual order for intravitreal ceftazidime 2.25 mg/0.1 mL. Your pharmacy has ceftazidime already in solution at 100 mg/mL. Using 1 mL of that ceftazidime, how many milliliters of sodium chloride 0.9% would you have to add in order to prepare the proper concentration?

8. The following pediatric prescription is received by the pharmacy, and the drug label shows the drug to be dispensed.

   ℞ clindamycin 285 mg PO q8h

   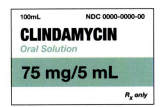

   a. What are the correct dosing instructions, in milliliters, for the dispensed label?

   _____

   b. How many doses are in the bottle shown in the label?

   _____

9. You receive an order for 1,200,000 units of penicillin G for a pediatric patient, and the drug label shows the solution available in stock. How many milliliters will provide the dose required?

   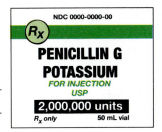

   _____
   _____

10. You receive the following prescription.

    ℞ Macrobid 100 mg PO bid x 14 days

    a. How should the dosing instructions on the dispensed label read?

    _____

    b. How many 100 mg capsules will be needed for a two-week supply?

    _____

UNDERSTANDING THE LARGER MEDICAL CONTEXT

1. While working in the hospital pharmacy, you receive the following medication order.

   ℞ Penicillamine 500 mg q6h for infected gums

   a. Is this drug appropriate to treat this infection? Why or why not?

   _____
   _____

   b. What alternatives might be more appropriate?

   _____
   _____

2. Timmy Thompson is a 13-year-old boy who has severe acne. He is the star right fielder for his Little League team and intends to spend most of his summer outside, playing baseball. His doctor writes the following prescription for Timmy's acne.

> **R$_x$** minocycline 100 mg PO daily

   a. What would you warn Timmy's parents about when they pick up the medication? Other than discontinuing the medication, how could this side effect be managed?

   _____
   _____

   b. How should Timmy limit his diet while taking this medication?

   _____
   _____

3. A patient in the ICU has been diagnosed with methicillin-resistant *S. aureus* in her blood. The drug chosen by the physician to treat this patient is Synercid. You overheard the physician say that he wants to use Synercid because the patient got severe flushing when she received vancomycin last year. He also mentioned that she received 1 g of vancomycin over 35 minutes. The order received reads as follows.

> **R$_x$** Synercid 600 mg IV q8h

   a. What solution should this medication be mixed in and why?

   _____
   _____

   b. What are two alternatives to Synercid for this patient?

   _____
   _____

4. Mr. Marshall calls your pharmacy because he misplaced his glasses and can't read the directions that accompanied his new Z-PAK prescription. On the phone, he says, "Let's see, I have six tablets here. Should I take them all at once, or will one a day be fine? I would also like to know if I should take this drug with my other medications before I go to bed." What are the instructions Mr. Marshall needs to take his Z-PAK?

   _____
   _____
   _____

5. Mr. Cowell has been on vancomycin 1500 mg IV q12h for a sternal wound infection for five days. His most recent trough came back at 22.5 mcg/mL (normal troughs are 10 mcg/mL to 15 mcg/mL), and was drawn appropriately. What would you expect to happen to his dose?

6. Mrs. Whang has been on Unasyn 1.5 g IV q6h for treatment of an infected cat bite. She is being discharged home. What oral antibiotic would give her an identical antimicrobial coverage?

7. Mr. Allen has been started on Vancocin 250 mg PO q6h. What do you think he is being treated for?

8. Mr. Mitchell has been on cefepime 2 g IV q8h for the treatment of *Pseuedomonas aeruginosa* (PA). When double covering PA, you need to use two different mechanisms of action to treat the infection. Here are the following sensitivities for Mr. Mitchell's PA infection:

   Sensitive: cefepime, Zosyn, amikacin

   Resistant: gentamicin, Cipro, Fortaz

   What do you think would be the best agent to treat Mr. Mitchell's PA? Why?

9. Dr. Hoar is a pharmacist who loves to quiz pharmacy technicians about their knowledge of antibiotics. When he spots you at the grocery store, he approaches you and asks, "What is the only fourth-generation cephalosporin?" What is your answer?

10. What medication with no antimicrobial activity is sometimes used in septic patients?

COMMUNICATING IN THE PHARMACY

1. A 45-year-old woman brings in a prescription for tetracycline 250 mg PO q6h. What are three important counseling points for this medication, and what are some appropriate auxiliary labels to place on the prescription vial?

2. A nurse from a doctor's office attempts to call in a prescription to your retail pharmacy. She requests oxacillin 1 g every six hours. What would your reply be?

_____
_____

3. A unit in your hospital only has dialysis patients. You are working in the IV room when you receive an order for Levaquin 500 mg IV q24h. What about that dose would you bring to the pharmacist's attention?

_____

4. You receive a label in your IV room for Bactrim 210 mg. You have no idea if it is for a pediatric or adult patient. What question should you ask the pharmacist?

_____

5. A patient calls the pharmacy and says, "I have some Keflex liquid left over from my son, can I start using it for my daughter?" What should the patient be told?

_____

DISPENSING AND STORING DRUGS

Where or how should the following medications be stored in the pharmacy?

1. Amoxil suspension before reconstitution

   _____

2. amoxicillin-clavulanate suspension after reconstitution

   _____

3. Bactrim suspension

   _____

4. metronidazole tablets

   _____

5. quinupristin-dalfopristin injection before reconstitution

   _____

6. Synercid injection after reconstitution

   _____

7. Xigris vials

   _____

8. Tequin tablets

   _____

9. reconstituted cefoxitin
   _____

10. clindamycin oral solution
    _____

What auxiliary labels would you put on the following medications?

11. metronidazole tablets
    _____

12. Levaquin tablets
    _____

13. Dynabac tablets
    _____

14. Ketek
    _____

15. Gantrisin
    _____

PUTTING SAFETY FIRST

Do the doses match the medications? If not, give a common dose.

1. Cipro 500 mg IV daily
   _____

2. vancomycin 1000 mg PO bid
   _____

3. minocycline 100 mg PO bid
   _____

4. Augmentin suspension 125 mg/5 mL, 1 tsp PO tid
   _____

5. cefazolin 500 mg PO q6h
   _____

6. Primaxin 500 mg IV q6h
   _____

Identify the following drug interactions.

7. Name at least four drugs from at least two different classes that may have their effectiveness decreased with antacid use.

   _____

   _____

8. Name a drug that will interact with neuromuscular blockers and, as a result, will have increased toxicity.

   _____

9. Name a drug that should not be taken with atorvastatin.

   _____

10. Describe the interaction between metronidazole and alcohol-containing compounds.

    _____

PUZZLING THE TECHNICIAN

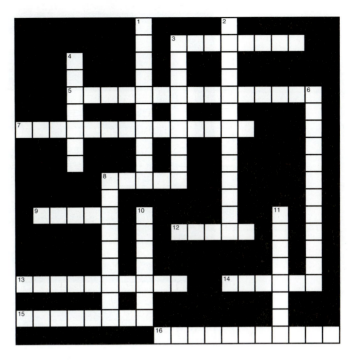

Across

3. only fourth-generation cephalosporin
5. class of antibiotics that can cause the patient to be at risk for nephrotoxicity and ototoxicity
7. bactericidal agent that inhibits the infecting organism from multiplying
8. brand name of an extended-spectrum penicillin combined with a beta-lactamase inhibitor
9. generation of cephalosporins that contains Ancef and cephalexin
12. antimicrobial related to the macrolides and known to cause blurred vision
13. only medication able to treat methicillin-resistant *S. aureus* (MRSA) in the blood
14. also known as Activated Protein C
15. broad-spectrum antibiotic with the potential to cause seizures when used in high doses or in patients with renal disease
16. agent for PCP pneumonia in patients allergic to sulfonamides

Down

1. medication class that contains ciprofloxacin, levofloxacin, and gatifloxacin
2. drug that has the potential to cause nausea and vomiting
3. process in which calcium will interfere with the absorption of tetracyclines, thus decreasing their efficacy
4. monobactam considered safe to use in a patient with severe penicillin allergy
6. oldest class of antimicrobial agents
8. brand name for a type of macrolide that can treat a variety of infections with a single loading dose of 500 mg, followed by four days of 250 mg
10. agent for dental prophylaxis in patients with an allergic history to penicillin
11. brand-name drug for quinupristin-dalfopristin

PUZZLING TERMINOLOGY

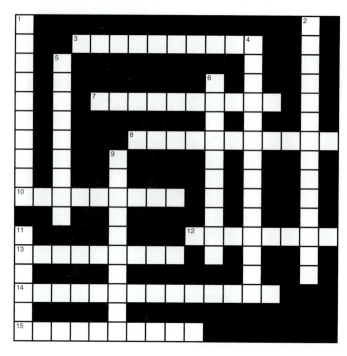

Across

3. a class of antibiotics that inhibit protein synthesis by combining with ribosomes; used primarily to treat pulmonary infections caused by Legionella and gram-positive organisms
7. a class of antibiotics with rapid bactericidal action against most gram-negative and many gram-positive bacteria; work by causing DNA breakage and cell death; cross the blood-brain barrier
8. damaging the organs of hearing
10. combination with a metal in complexes in which the metal is part of a ring
12. microorganisms that cause infection
13. treatment begun before a definite diagnosis
14. a class of antibiotics that inhibit protein synthesis within the bacterial ribosomes; useful in the treatment of vancomycin- and methicillin-resistant infections
15. a systemic disease associated with pathogenic microorganisms or their toxins in the blood; often called blood poisoning

Down

1. a substance that inhibits the growth of microorganisms without killing them
2. destructive to the kidneys
4. a new infection complicating the course of therapy of an existing infection
5. a class of antibiotics that block protein synthesis by binding to ribosomal subunits and may also inhibit the formation of newly forming ribosomes; used primarily to treat bacterial infections in the lungs and sinuses
6. infections acquired by patients when they are in the hospital
9. a chemical substance with the ability to kill or inhibit the growth of organisms by interfering with bacteria life processes
11. a systemic inflammatory response to infection resulting from blood-borne infections

Therapy for Fungi and Viruses

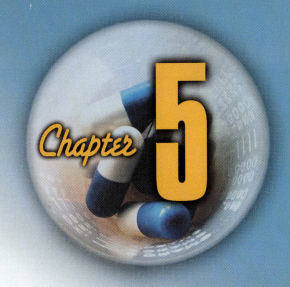

Chapter 5

READING DRUG LABELS AND MEDICATION ORDERS

1. You are presented with the following prescription, and the drug label shown is the product you pick up from the pharmacy shelf.

    amphotericin B 60 mg IV in NS over 4 hours for 7 days

   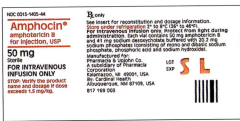

   Reproduced with permission of Pfizer Inc. All rights reserved.

   a. Is normal saline an appropriate diluent for amphotericin? If not, why?

   _____

   b. Assuming the patient receives the full seven days of therapy, how many total grams will be administered? Show your calculation.

   _____

   c. How many vials should you have on hand to last the seven days? Explain your answer.

   _____
   _____

2. You are presented with the following prescription, and the drug label shown is the product available in the pharmacy.

    Valtrex (valacyclovir) 1 g PO bid x 10 days

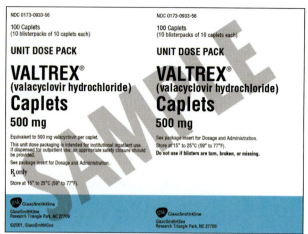

For educational use only. Reproduced with permission of GlaxoSmithKline.

    a. How many caplets will you dispense? Explain your answer.

    _____

    _____

    b. How will the instructions read on the label?

    _____

    _____

3. Ms. Blake brings in the following prescription for her son Joey. Because Joey cannot swallow tablets, she asks you to fill the prescription with a liquid form. You have amantadine syrup 50 mg/5 mL in stock. (*Note:* 1 tsp = 5 mL. This and other equivalencies are available in the Pharmacy Library section of the IRC for this title at www.emcp.com.)

    ℞ amantadine 100 mg PO bid x 3 days

    a. How many milliliters are in one dose?

    _____

    b. How many teaspoonsful are in one dose?

    _____

    c. How will the instructions read on the prescription label?

    _____

    _____

    d. How many milliliters will you dispense?

    _____

4. The following order is received by the hospital pharmacy for a patient who weighs 84 lb. (*Note:* 1 kg = 2.2 lb. This and other equivalencies are available in the Pharmacy Library section of the IRC for this title at www.emcp.com.)

> ℞ acyclovir 10 mg/kg IV q8h

a. What would be the total amount of acyclovir per dose?

b. Provided that you have a 50 mg/mL vial, how many milliliters would you be using per day?

c. The maximum concentration for acyclovir to be infused is 7 mg/mL. What is the minimum volume to administer this dose? Use the the intravenous solutions available commercially (50 mL, 100 mL, 150 mL, 250 mL, 500 mL, and 1000 mL).

5. What is wrong with the following prescription?

> ℞ Fuzeon (enfuvirtide) 90 mg PO bid

6. You receive the following prescription, and the drug label shows the product available.

> ℞ Videx (didanosine) suspension 100 mg PO bid

a. How would you reconstitute the powder in the bottle?

b. What volume of didanosine liquid would the patient take per day?

c. Assuming the dose does not change, how many days will a 200 mL bottle last?

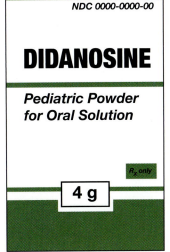

NDC 0000-0000-00

DIDANOSINE

Pediatric Powder for Oral Solution

℞ only

4 g

7. You receive the following prescription.

   ℞ Relenza 75 mg PO bid

   a. What is wrong with this prescription?
   _____

   b. What do you think the intended drug was?
   _____

   c. What auxiliary label would you affix to the prescription vial?
   _____

8. You receive the following prescription, and the drug label indicates the drug is available as 250 mg capsules.

   ℞ ganciclovir 500 mg PO bid

   a. Using the drug indicated by the label, calculate how many capsules would be required for a month's supply.
   _____

   b. What other dosage forms are there for ganciclovir?
   _____

9. You receive the following prescription.

   ℞ saquinavir 600 mg PO tid on an empty stomach

   a. Which brand-name product is the patient most likely taking? Why?
   _____

   b. What auxiliary labels would you affix to the prescription vial?
   _____

10. You receive the following prescription, and the drug label shown is the medication available in the pharmacy.

> **Rx** nystatin 1 tsp swish and swallow 4 times daily

a. How long will the bottle last if no doses are missed? Show your calculation.

_____
_____
_____
_____

b. If the patient is to receive therapy for one week, how many bottles would you dispense? Show your calculation.

_____
_____
_____
_____

Label: 60mL NDC 0000-0000-00
100,000 units per mL
NYSTATIN
ORAL SUSPENSION USP
Shake well before using
Caution: Federal law prohibits dispensing without prescription

UNDERSTANDING THE LARGER MEDICAL CONTEXT

1. Mr. Tolman, a patient at your pharmacy, has been having problems with oral candidiasis since he started his radiation therapy. His doctor has given him nystatin swish and swallow without improvement for one week. What alternatives might be prescribed for Mr. Tolman?

_____

2. Ms. Benitez has been on conventional amphotericin B therapy for broad-spectrum, antifungal infection for three days. Her signs of infection have been improving; however, today her labs arrive, suggesting that the amphotericin is toxic to her kidneys. Since she has been doing well on amphotericin B from a treatment perspective, what alternatives could treat her infection?

_____

3. Mrs. Bentley is an elderly woman who has trouble remembering when to take her medicine. She has just been discharged with the prescription acyclovir 800 mg PO five times daily for seven days for herpes zoster.

   a. Mrs. Bentley is concerned that she will forget to take 35 doses of medication. Which medication could be substituted for acyclovir?

   _____

   b. What doses would you expect to see, assuming she has no liver or kidney problems?

   _____
   _____

4. A Parkinson's patient comes into the pharmacy with a prescription for Tamiflu 75 mg PO bid. You notice that he has been on Symmetrel 100 mg PO bid for the past six months.

   a. What type of influenza virus do you think the patient has contracted? Why?

   b. How long should this patient take the Tamiflu?

5. Mr. Daniels is an HIV patient of yours who has been known to abuse alcohol. Which HIV medications would you *not* expect Mr. Daniels to be able to take?

6. Miss Harvey comes into your pharmacy feeling nauseous. She is short of breath and has abdominal pain and a rash on her chest. You know that she recently started a new HIV regimen because her old regimen was no longer effective in reducing her viral load. You call 911 for her. While the EMTs are stabilizing her, they ask the pharmacist what medications she is taking that might cause these reactions.

   a. What three antiretrovirals have been known to cause hypersensitivity allergic reactions?

   b. You look in Miss Harvey's profile and see that she has been taking Bactrim for PCP prophylaxis and glyburide (a sulfonamide) for her diabetes. Given her medication history and the fact that she has no swelling of the throat or lips, which antiretroviral do you think she may have started?

7. Mr. Dellenbach has been on his current investigational drug regimen of Sustiva, Kaletra, emtricitabine, and stavudine for the past year. Because of nightmares, the Sustiva will be switched to either Viramune or Rescriptor. How might each drug interact with his current drug regimen?

8. Mrs. Faragon is an HIV patient who believes in taking as many vitamin supplements as possible to stay healthy. She currently takes a fat-soluble supervitamin that provides 300% of her recommended daily allowance for vitamins A, D, and E. With which antiretroviral would this be a potential problem? Why?

9. Nurse Ratchet, an emergency room nurse, suffered a needle-stick injury when caring for an HIV patient who was in a motor vehicle accident. What medications would you expect her to start? What would the dosing regimen be for each drug?

10. Mr. Cruz has been in the hospital for seven days. During his hospital stay, he has been on broad-spectrum antimicrobials, and three days ago he started amphotericin B. He is still presenting with signs of infection, without improvement. Viral causes have been ruled out.

   a. What other antifungal might be prescribed for Mr. Cruz?

   b. The doctor receives culture results for the fungal infection, and decides to start Vfend. How will that drug be dosed?

COMMUNICATING IN THE PHARMACY

1. While working in a hospital sterile products room, you get a label to make foscarnet 7000 mg IV q12h. For the benefit of a new pharmacy technician, identify other intravenous items you would expect to prepare for this patient.

2. While working in a hospital sterile products room, you get a label to make amphotericin B 75 mg IV. Explain to a new pharmacy technician what premedications you would expect to prepare before sending the amphotericin B.

3. A patient in the ICU has uncontrolled blood sugars. A request has been made to change the patient's Abelcet from D_5W to 0.9% sodium chloride. Explain to the ICU staff what the problem is with this request.

4. Mr. Hatcher has been HIV-positive for six years. He comes into your pharmacy to get his new prescription regimen, which includes Kaletra, Sustiva, and Norvir. What potential problem do you bring to the pharmacist's attention?

DISPENSING AND STORING DRUGS

1. Which NNRTIs require that a patient avoid antacids?

2. With which antiviral should you use chemotherapeutic precautions?

3. Which antivirals are available in both intravenous and by-mouth dosage forms?

4. Which NNRTI has been shown to decrease the effectiveness of oral contraceptives?

5. Which NRTI should be stored in an airtight container?

6. Which HIV medication should be dispensed with alcohol pads to clean the injection site before administration?

7. Which auxiliary label would you place on an itraconazole prescription?

8. On which antifungals would you affix a "For external use only" label?

9. Which antiviral would a pharmacy stock, but never dispense directly to a patient?

10. Which auxiliary label should accompany Ziagen (abacavir)?

11. How would you store Cancidas (caspofungin) vials before reconstitution?

12. How would you store any amphotericin B formulation before reconstitution?

13. What three auxiliary labels should be affixed to a Crixivan (indinavir) prescription?

14. Which NRTIs should have a "Do not take with alcoholic beverages" auxiliary label?

15. Which protease inhibitor should have an "Avoid exposure to sunlight" auxiliary label?

PUTTING SAFETY FIRST

Does the requested dose match the typical medication dose in the following orders? If not, provide the typical dosage for each medication.

1. Lamisil 250 mg PO bid
   _____

2. fluconazole 100 mg tid
   _____

3. caspofungin 50 mg IV daily
   _____

4. rimantadine 150 mg PO bid
   _____

5. amphotericin B 2 g IV daily
   _____

6. valganciclovir 900 mg PO bid
   _____

7. famciclovir 200 mg PO five times daily for genital herpes outbreak
   _____

8. Videx EC 400 mg PO qam ac
   _____

9. Where would you store a dose of intravenous acyclovir after it has already been made?
   _____

10. You have a patient who has been on the following regimen for HIV:

    Sustiva 600 mg PO daily

    Epivir 150 mg PO bid

    Agenerase 1200 mg PO tid

    Ritonavir 200 mg bid has been added by the patient's physician. What dose in the patient's HIV regimen would you expect will change and why?
    _____
    _____

Name _____ Date _____

PUZZLING THE TECHNICIAN

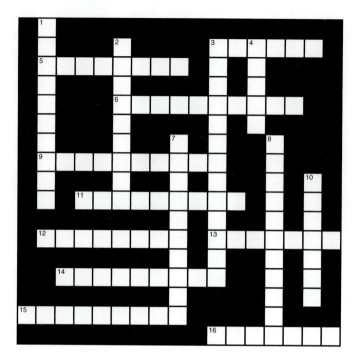

Across

3. only HIV medication *not* used orally
5. only glucan synthesis inhibitor
6. antiviral used for Parkinson's disease
9. brand name for delaviridine
11. non-liposomal version of amphotericin
12. antifungal available intravenously as well as orally
13. brand name for valacyclovir
14. drug that Valtrex gets converted to
15. only nucleotide reverse transcriptase inhibitor
16. combination brand-name drug that contains lopinavir and ritonavir

Down

1. topical antifungal used for onychomycosis and applied at bedtime
2. used primarily in respiratory syncytial virus
3. prodrug for amprenavir with fewer GI side effects
4. NRTI known to cause pancreatitis and peripheral neurophathy
7. generic name for Reyataz
8. used with amphotericin B for *Candida* or *Cryptococcus*
10. inhalational antiviral used for influenza

PUZZLING TERMINOLOGY

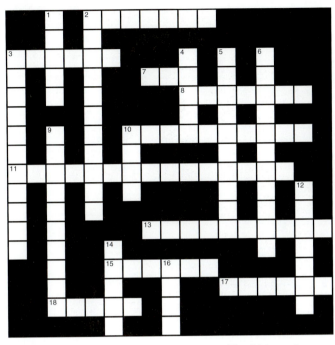

Across

2. a viral infection that has a protracted course with long periods of remission interspersed with recurrence
3. an individual viral particle capable of infecting a living cell; consists of nucleic acid surrounded by a capsid (protein shell)
7. a common viral infection; influenza
8. the ability of a virus to lie dormant and then, under certain conditions, reproduce and again behave like an infective agent, causing cell damage
10. a virus without an envelope covering the capsid
11. drugs that limit the progression of HIV
13. a form of lipid found in the cell membrane of fungi
15. a protein shell that surrounds and protects the nucleic acid within a virus particle
17. a single-cell organism similar to a human cell; marked by the absence of chlorophyll, a rigid cell wall, and reproduction by spores
18. a drug that inhibits HIV reverse transcriptase by competing with natural nucleic acid substrates, causing termination of chain formation

Down

1. a drug that inhibits HIV reverse transcriptase at a different site than an NRTI targets
2. a eukaryotic sterol that in higher animals is the precursor of bile acids and steroid hormones and a key constituent of cell membranes
3. the introduction of a vaccine, a component of an infectious agent, into the body to produce immunity to the actual agent
4. a regimen of dosing one week per month; commonly used for treating fungal nail infections
5. agents that prevent virus replication in a host cell without interfering with the host's normal function
6. a viral infection that spreads to other tissues by way of the bloodstream or the central nervous system
9. a substance that exerts virus-nonspecific but host-specific antiviral activity by inducing gene coding for antiviral proteins that inhibit the synthesis of viral RNA
10. a drug that inhibits HIV reverse transcriptase, to prevent the formation of RNA from proviral DNA causing a decrease in the amount of virus in the body and subsequent spread to other healthy cells
12. a compound that on administration and chemical conversion by metabolic processes becomes an active pharmacological agent
14. a viral infection that quickly resolves with no latent infection
16. a viral infection that maintains a progressive course over months or years with cumulative damage to body tissues, ultimately ending in the host's death

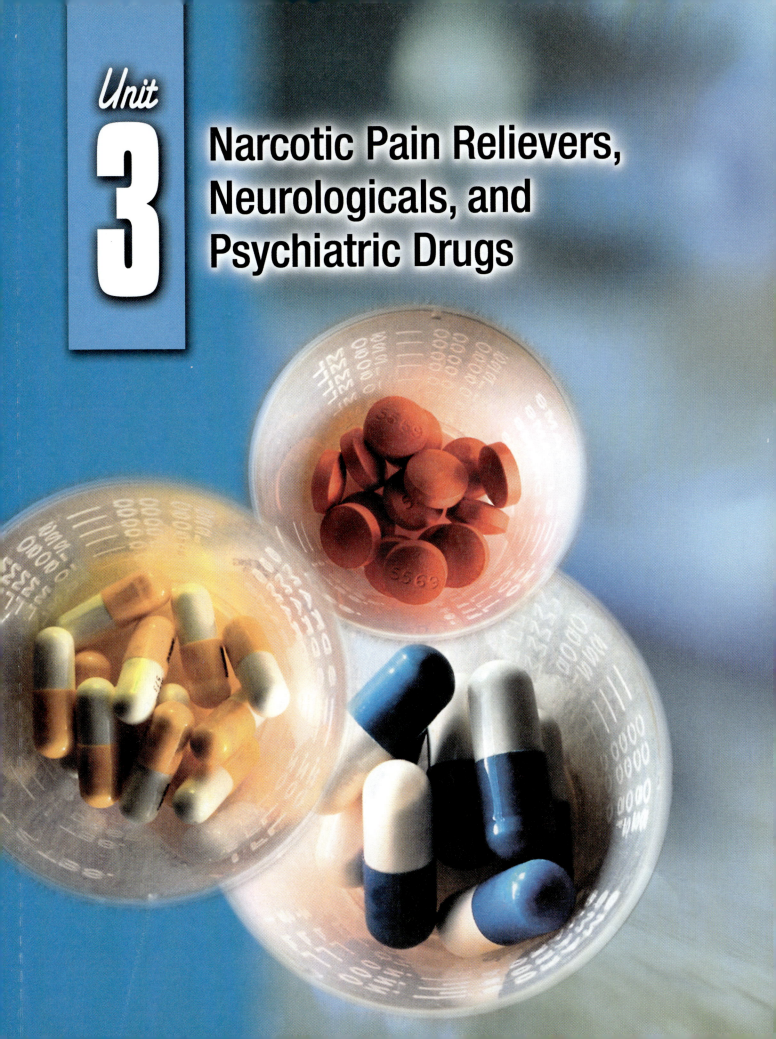

Unit 3
Narcotic Pain Relievers, Neurologicals, and Psychiatric Drugs

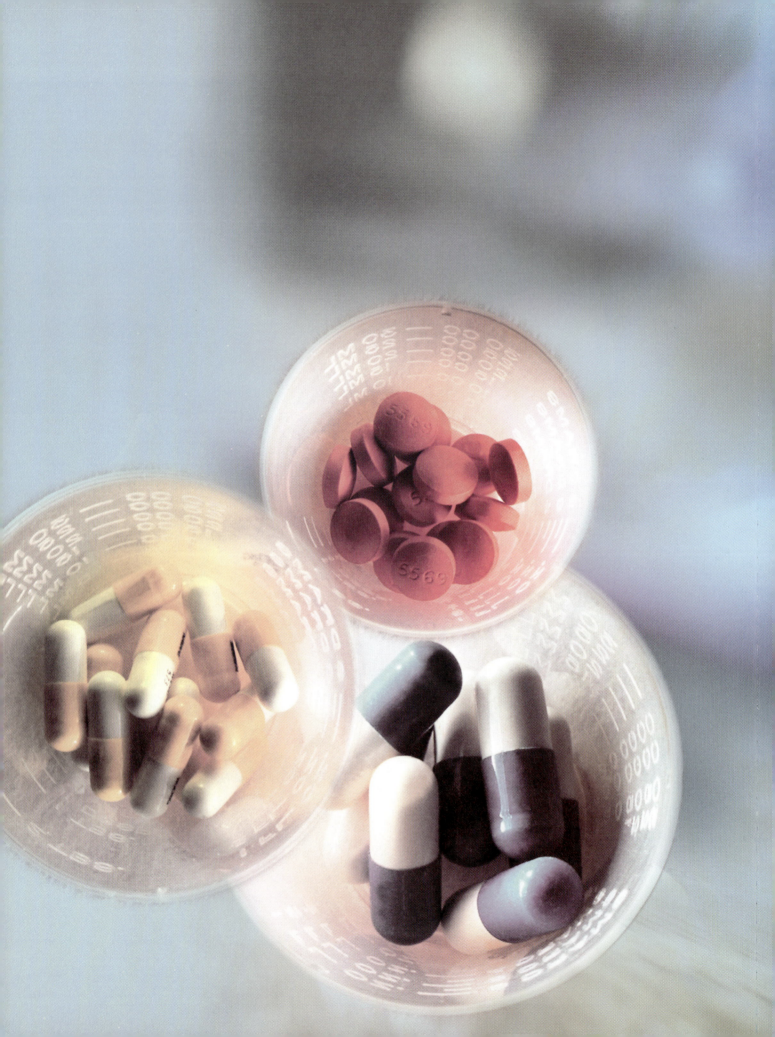

Anesthetics, Analgesics, and Narcotics

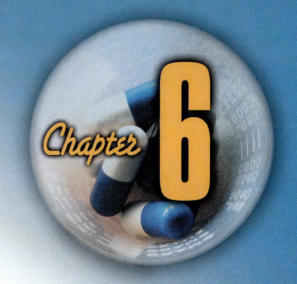

Chapter 6

READING DRUG LABELS AND MEDICATION ORDERS

1. You receive the following prescription, and you identify the label shown as the corresponding product available in the pharmacy.

   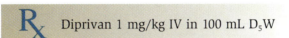

   ℞ Diprivan 1 mg/kg IV in 100 mL D$_5$W

   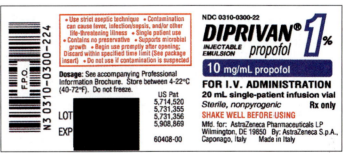

   Used with permission of AstraZeneca.

   a. Is this okay to prepare as written? If not, why?

   b. The patient's chart indicates that the patient is 175 lb. How much Diprivan is needed?

   c. How many milliliters of the product shown in the label will be used?

2. In the outpatient pharmacy, you receive the following prescription.

   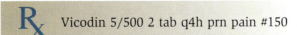

   ℞ Vicodin 5/500 2 tab q4h prn pain #150

   a. Is this prescription okay to dispense as is? If not, why?

b. If the patient takes the prescription as written, what would the total daily dose of acetaminophen be?

c. What other product might the pharmacist recommend to the prescriber?

3. While working at an inpatient pharmacy, you notice Nimbex 2 mg/mL on the shelf.

   a. What is the generic name?

   b. How many milligrams of the active ingredient are in each 10 mL vial?

   c. Where should this medication be stored in the pharmacy?

UNDERSTANDING THE LARGER MEDICAL CONTEXT

1. You work in a children's hospital and notice many inhaled anesthetics except desflurane. Why is desflurane not available?

2. A doctor calls your pharmacy and asks if Buprenex should be taken on a full or empty stomach. What is the correct answer?

3. A nurse calls from one of the floors and asks what strengths of Percocet are available. What are they?

4. Which class of local anesthetic should be avoided in patients with liver insufficiency?

5. Is ketamine (Ketalar) an appropriate anesthetic for a patient with uncontrolled hypertension? Why or why not?

6. Does the autonomic nervous system regulate body systems under voluntary or involuntary control?

7. What are the five components of a classic migraine headache?

8. What class of drug is eletriptan (Relpax) in?

9. What dosage forms are commercially available for metoclopramide (Reglan)?

10. Why would you find flumazenil (Romazicon) in an emergency room kit? What are possible side effects of this drug?

11. A doctor calls and is looking for a sublingual tablet for migraines but not the "ergot" one. What drug is she looking for?

COMMUNICATING IN THE PHARMACY

1. Mr. Patel comes into your pharmacy for a refill of his Stadol NS. He jokes, "I only get a few squirts, and then it's empty." What should you tell Mr. Patel about his prescription?

2. As Mr. Jones is picking up his prescription for Demerol (meperidine), he tells you that his doctor recommended he take an over-the-counter laxative. He wants to know which one he should take. What do you think the pharmacist will recommend? Explain your answer.

3. A patient brings in the following prescription. What is important to tell the patient about these directions?

> **Rx** Zomig 5 mg tablet, 1 tab at onset of headache. May repeat prn.

_____
_____
_____
_____

4. When picking up his refill for Midrin, Mr. Neilson tells you that his migraines are so bad, they sometimes make his fingers go numb. How should you respond to Mr. Neilson?

_____
_____
_____
_____

5. As you are reviewing a prescription for propranolol with a patient, the patient sees on the package insert that the drug is used to control blood pressure. The patient becomes irate, and tells you that the prescription is wrong. She was to get something for her headaches, and she wants you to contact the doctor immediately. What do you say?

_____
_____
_____
_____

DISPENSING AND STORING DRUGS

Where should the following medication be stored? Indicate an answer for both in the pharmacy and in the patient's home.

1. mivacurium (Mivacron)

   _____

2. atracurium (Tacrium)

   _____

3. calcitonin

   _____
   _____

4. succinylcholine
   _____

5. Stadol Nasal Spray
   _____

What auxiliary labels would you put on the following medication?
6. morphine
   _____
   _____

7. propofol
   _____
   _____
   _____

8. eletriptan (Relpax)
   _____

9. metoclopramide
   _____

10. naloxone
    _____

11. A patient walks into the pharmacy and wants to know if the FDA has approved any OTC migraine medications. If there is a product, what are the active ingredients? (Use the FDA Web site at www.fda.gov.)
    _____
    _____
    _____
    _____

12. What is the maximum weekly dosage of cafergot 2 mg suppository? (Use the drug package insert, Drug Facts and Comparisons, or the FDA Web site at www.fda.gov.)
    _____
    _____

Name _____ Date _____

PUTTING SAFETY FIRST

Does the requested dose match the typical medication dose in the following orders? If not, provide the typical dosage for each medication.

1. Percocet 6/325 1 tab tid prn

2. Imitrex tablets 50 mg, 1 tab at onset of headache, may repeat in 30 minutes prn

3. Imitrex 6 mg INJ, 6 mg SC at onset of headache, may repeat in one hour prn. NTE 2 INJ (12 mg/24 hours)

4. Hydrocodone 5/500, 2 tabs q4h prn

5. Duragesic 25 mcg/hour, apply 1 patch every day

PUZZLING THE TECHNICIAN

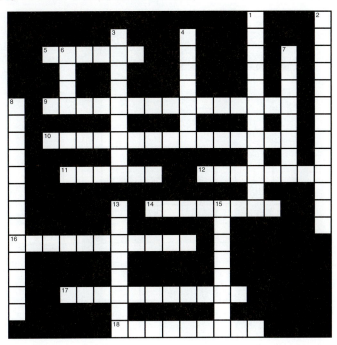

Across

5. brand name of pentazocine
9. effect of epinephrine when administered with a local anesthetic
10. neuromuscular blocking agent that works by depolarizing mechanism
11. class of short-acting local anesthetics
12. generic name for Duragesic
14. drug that causes associative amnesia
16. drug of choice for prophylactic migraine treatment
17. generic for Carbocaine
18. benzodiazepine with the fastest onset of action

Down

1. selective 5-HT receptor agonist with maximum of 10 mg/day
2. neurotransmitter that acts on smooth and cardiac muscle
3. OTC amide anesthetic
4. part of the peripheral nervous system that regulates smooth muscle
6. sensation that precedes a migraine—visual disturbance
7. doses in a container of Stadol NS
8. drug used to treat addiction
13. brand name of the drug used to treat malignant hyperthermia
15. brand name of nasal spray containing ergotamine

PUZZLING TERMINOLOGY

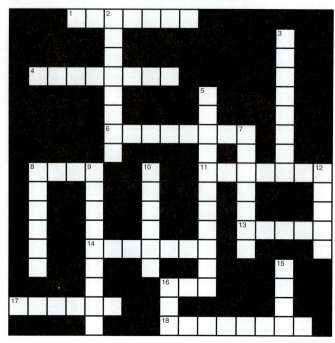

Across

1. the part of the efferent system of the PNS that regulates the skeletal muscles
4. the nerves that dispatch information out from the CNS; part of the peripheral nervous system
6. a pain-modulating chemical derived from opium or synthetically produced
8. a subjective sensation or motor phenomenon that precedes and marks the onset of a migraine headache
11. the type of anesthesia used to produce a condition characterized by reversible unconsciousness, analgesia, skeletal muscle relaxation, and amnesia on recovery
13. nerve receptors that control vasoconstriction, pupil dilation, and relaxation of the GI smooth muscle
14. nerve cells
16. the nerves and sense organs outside the CNS
17. any narcotic that has opiate-like activity, i.e., insensibility or stupor
18. the nerves and sense organs that bring information to the CNS; part of the peripheral nervous system

Down

2. a severe, throbbing, vascular headache, usually resulting in nausea, photophobia, phonophobia, and hyperesthesia
3. a theory that proposes that migraine headaches are caused by vasodilation and the concomitant mechanical stimulation of sensory nerve endings
5. drugs used to reverse benzodiazepine or narcotic overdoses
7. the part of the nervous system consisting of the brain and spinal cord
8. a longer-acting class of local anesthetics that are metabolized by liver enzymes
9. the part of the efferent system of the PNS that regulates activities of body structures not under voluntary control
10. a short-acting class of local anesthetics, metabolized by pseudocholinesterase of the plasma and tissue fluids
12. the type of anesthesia used to produce a transient and reversible loss of sensation in a defined area of the body
15. a protective signal to warn of damage or presence of disease; the fifth vital sign
16. pain control whereby the patient can regulate, within certain limits, the administration of pain medication through a pump

Antidepressants, Antipsychotics, Antianxiety Agents, and Alcoholism

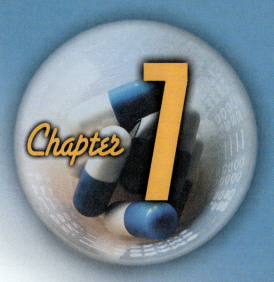

Chapter 7

READING DRUG LABELS AND MEDICATION ORDERS

1. You receive a prescription that indicates the patient is to take "500 mg qam for 10 days." The medication is available in 250 mg tablets.

   a. How many tablets will the patient take in a day?

   b. How many tablets will be dispensed?

2. You receive the following prescription, and you identify Desyrel 100 mg tablets as the corresponding product available in the pharmacy.

   ℞ Desyrel 75 mg daily disp 1 mo supply

   a. The patient insists on getting this prescription from your pharmacy today, so the only option is to dispense the available product. How can the patient administer the available tablets to get the correct dosage?

   b. How many tablets need to be dispensed?

   c. At what time of day should the patient take this medication and why?

3. You receive the following prescription, and you have Haldol 2 mg/mL available in the pharmacy.

   ℞ Haldol Liq 7 mg PO bid in 6 oz H_2O

a. How much liquid will constitute one dose?

b. How much product will need to be dispensed for a 30-day supply?

4. You receive the following prescription, and you identify the label shown as the corresponding product available in the pharmacy.

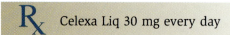
Rx Celexa Liq 30 mg every day

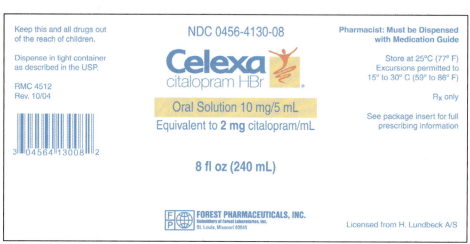
Reproduced with permission of Forest Laboratories, Inc.

a. How much liquid will be in each dose?

b. How long will the bottle last the patient?

UNDERSTANDING THE LARGER MEDICAL CONTEXT

1. What is the most common side effect of tricyclic antidepressants?

2. What side effect of some antipsychotic medications causes involuntary movements and may be irreversible?

3. Which type of anxiety can be controlled by minimizing outside stressors?

4. Why is clozapine not more commonly used?

5. What is the benefit of diphenhydramine over oxazepam for sleep disorders?

6. Which antidepressant works only on dopamine receptors?

7. Which would typically last longer, an anxiety attack or a panic attack? Explain your answer.

8. What are the major effects of long-term alcoholism on the body?

9. What is ECT?

10. A patient at your pharmacy knows not to take selegiline with foods containing tyramine, but she does not know which foods to avoid. Identify several foods containing tyramine she should avoid.

COMMUNICATING IN THE PHARMACY

1. While getting a refill of fluoxetine, Mrs. Adler mentions that she does not know why she is still taking it, as she has "felt fine for a while now." What do you say to her?

2. You noticed that Mr. Castrow was over a month late in refilling his prescription for Seroquel. You ask him why, and he says that he stopped taking it because it made him gain 15 lb. How do you help Mr. Castrow?

3. The hospital pharmacy receives an order for a cough syrup for a patient. The patient started taking disulfiram yesterday. What do you confirm about the cough syrup and why?

4. A patient brings back her prescription for Effexor to your pharmacy because she thinks the prescription was filled incorrectly. She has been taking the drug for over three weeks and does not feel any better. What should you tell her?

5. A dermatologist phones in a prescription for clindamycin for the treatment of acne for a patient. You notice in the profile that the patient has been on lithium for the last three months. Should you continue with the clindamycin prescription? Why or why not?

DISPENSING AND STORING DRUGS

1. What medication should you tell the patient not to take with soda?

2. Which SSRI usually does not cause drowsiness or somnolence?

3. Which class of medications is considered the safest for insomnia, in regard to side effects, dependence potential, and rebound insomnia?

4. With which drug will patients commonly self-medicate their anxiety or insomnia?

5. What are the effects of tardive dyskinesia?

What auxiliary labels would you put on the following medications?

6. zolpidem (Ambien)

7. carbamazepine (Tegretol XR)

8. desipramine

9. alprazolam

10. Depakote

Name   Date

What schedule are the following drugs?

11. chloral hydrate

12. secobarbital

13. zolpidem (Ambien)

14. diazepam

15. Recently the FDA made changes in the package insert of some antidepressants in the wake of pediatric and adolescent suicides. Using the FDA Web site (www.fda.gov), list at least 10 drugs that were affected.

PUTTING SAFETY FIRST

Does the requested dose match the typical medication dose in the following orders? If not, provide the typical dosage for each medication.

1. fluoxetine 25 mg bid

2. trazodone 100 mg hs prn

3. Ambien 5 mg hs #30

4. lithium 900 mg tid

5. Geodon 0.25 mg bid

6. Effexor XR 75 mg bid

7. bupropion SR 250 mg bid

8. Abilify 10 mg bid

9. Buspirone 10 mg every day

10. Paxil CR 25 mg every day

PUZZLING THE TECHNICIAN

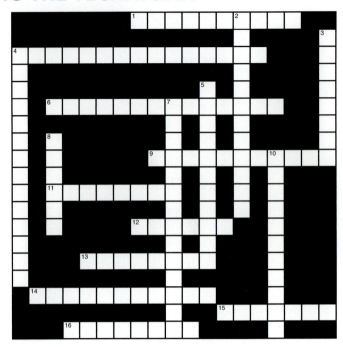

Across

1. drug approved for OCD, depression, and PMDD
4. serious side effect of clozapine
6. type of drug used in alcohol withdrawal to prevent delirium tremens
9. antidepressant commonly used in treating anorexia to stimulate weight gain
11. endocrine disorder linked to atypical antipsychotics
12. class of antidepressants that can be cardio-toxic
13. drug of choice for bipolar rapid cyclers
14. major side effect of tricyclic antidepressants, besides cardiotoxicity
15. naltrexone can be used to treat this addiction
16. reason for trazodone being avoided in males

Down

2. antipsychotic with a ceiling dose
3. name for type of reaction that includes nausea, severe vomiting, chest pain, thirst, and blurred vision
4. class of OTC agents useful in insomnia
5. drug commonly used to control extrapyramidal side effects
7. class of drugs associated with blindness from melanin deposits in the retina
8. atypical antipsychotic with low incidence of weight gain
10. beta blocker shown to be effective for migraine headaches and some types of anxiety

PUZZLING TERMINOLOGY

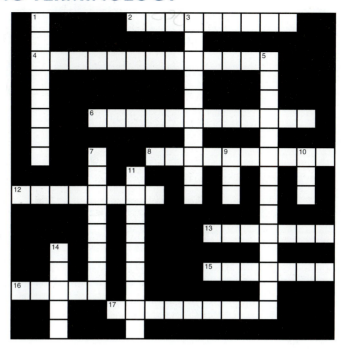

Across

2. drugs that induce sleep
4. a chronic psychotic disorder manifested by retreat from reality, delusions, hallucinations, ambivalence, withdrawal, and bizarre or regressive behavior
6. another term for antipsychotics
8. a condition characterized by the feeling that life has no meaning, pessimism, intense sadness, loss of concentration, and problems with eating and sleeping
12. major depression with no mania
13. a patient with this disorder presents with mood swings that alternate between periods of major depression and periods of mild-to-severe chronic agitation
15. a state of uneasiness characterized by apprehension and worry about possible events
16. a mood of extreme excitement, excessive elation, hyperactivity, agitation, and increased psychomotor activity
17. anxiety caused by factors outside the organism

Down

1. difficulty falling asleep or staying asleep or not feeling refreshed on awakening
3. a sleep disorder in which inappropriate attacks of sleep occur during the daytime hours
5. drugs that are used to treat schizophrenia; reduce symptoms of hallucinations, delusions, and thought disorders; also called neuroleptics
7. loss of appetite
9. the introduction of a brief but convulsive electrical stimulation through the brain; used as therapy for major depressive disorders
10. this disorder causes recurrent, persistent urges to perform repetitive acts such as hand washing
11. short periods of muscle weakness and loss of muscle tone associated with sudden emotions such as joy, fear, or anger; a symptom of narcolepsy
14. intense, overwhelming, and uncontrollable anxiety

Anticonvulsants and Drugs to Treat Other CNS Disorders

Chapter 8

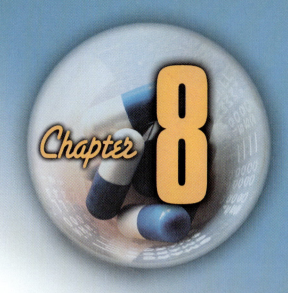

READING DRUG LABELS AND MEDICATION ORDERS

1. You receive the following prescription. What is the problem with the prescription as written?

   ℞ Clonazepam 0.5 mg 1 tid #90 refill x 11

   _____
   _____

2. You receive the following prescription, and the drug label shown is the product available in the pharmacy. How many tablets will you dispense? Show your calculation.

   ℞ Dilantin 50 mg bid x 2 days, then 50 mg qid x 8 days

   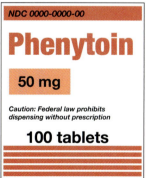

   _____
   _____
   _____

3. You receive the following prescription, and the drug label shown is the product available in the pharmacy.

   ℞ Sinemet CR 25/100 II q6am, 1/2 noon, I 1/2 4pm, II 8pm

   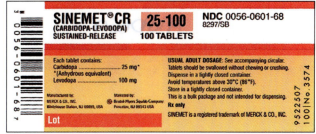

   Used with permission of Merck & Co., Inc.

a. Is this prescription okay to fill with the product shown?

yes.

b. How many tablets will be needed for a 30-day supply?

4. You receive the following order for a patient who weighs 88 kg. The pharmacy has the product shown in the following drug label.

Rx Imuran IV 1.75 mg/kg/day

AZATHIOPRINE SODIUM FOR INJECTION, USP
FOR IV USE ONLY
Equivalent to
100 mg
Azathioprine
Rx ONLY

NDC 55390-600-20   STERILE LYOPHILIZED MATERIAL
Usual Dose: See package insert.
Each vial contains azathioprine sodium, equivalent to 100 mg azathioprine, sodium hydroxide and, if necessary, hydrochloric acid to adjust pH.
Preparation of solution: Inject into the vial 10 mL Sterile Water for Injection.
Swirl the vial until a clear solution results. Use within 24 hours.
Store between 15° to 25° C (59° to 77° F).
Protect from light. Retain in carton until time of use.
Manufactured by: Manufactured for:
Ben Venue Laboratories, Inc.   Bedford Laboratories™
Bedford, OH 44146   Bedford, OH 44146   AZV03

Used with permission of Bedford Laboratories.

a. What is the daily dose going to be? Show your calculation.

b. Is this the correct product?

c. How much product would be used in a six-day supply? Show your calculation.

UNDERSTANDING THE LARGER MEDICAL CONTEXT

1. What are the different types of generalized seizures?

Tonic-clonic, absence, myoclonic, and atonic.

2. Loss of dopaminergic neurons from which region of the brain leads to Parkinson's disease?

Midbrain.

3. What is the benefit of levodopa-carbidopa over levodopa alone?

   It is much more smoother, more rapid induction into therapy with this drug.

4. What is the most common reason for drug therapy failure in epilepsy?

   The side effects of the drug they use.

5. What is the first-line treatment(s) and route of administration for *status epilepticus*?

6. What is the drug of choice for a patient who begins to seize after severe head trauma?

7. What are signs and symptoms of myasthenia gravis?

8. What are the three hallmark characteristics of attention-deficit hyperactivity disorder?

9. How does multiple sclerosis affect muscle use?

10. Which disease is the result of amyloid plaque forming in the brain?

COMMUNICATING IN THE PHARMACY

1. Mr. Roberts arrives at the pharmacy with a new prescription for Eldepryl. His doctor told him that because Eldepryl is an MAOI-type drug, he cannot eat cheese or have any alcohol while taking this drug. What might the pharmacist tell Mr. Roberts?

   _____
   _____
   _____
   _____

2. Mrs. Simon arrives at the pharmacy on a Friday afternoon to refill her ethosuximide (Zarontin), as she took her last dose that morning. You have none in stock and will not receive any until Monday. Can the patient wait? What should you do?

   _____
   _____
   _____
   _____

3. A nurse calls from one of the floors in the hospital and wants you to add a phenobarbital allergy to a profile. She says that the patient developed a rash. She is waiting for the doctor to see the patient, but she wants to know what else the pharmacy carries for the seizure type treated with phenobarbital.

   _____
   _____
   _____
   _____

4. What can you tell a patient about phenytoin side effects? What can be done to prevent those side effects? What warnings should you give the patient about this drug?

   _____
   _____
   _____
   _____

5. What can you tell a patient about starting on the drug Avonex?

   _____
   _____
   _____

DISPENSING AND STORING DRUGS

Where or how should the following medications be stored in the pharmacy?

1. glatiramer acetate (Copaxone)

2. phenytoin suspension

3. methylphenidate

4. interferon beta-1a (Avonex)

5. donepezil (Aricept)

What auxiliary labels would you put on the following medications?

6. zonisamide (Zonegran)

7. methylphenidate (Concerta)

8. rivastigmine (Exelon)

9. tacrine (Cognex)

10. interferon beta-1a (Avonex)

11. Your pharmacist wants you to use MedlinePlus to find information about ginkgo biloba use in Alzheimer's patients. She wants to know if any clinical trials are being performed. What do you find out?

Name   Date

PUTTING SAFETY FIRST

Does the requested dose match the typical medication dose in the following orders? If not, provide the typical dosage for each medication.

1. Sinemet 25/100 qid

2. Zonegran 200 mg bid

3. neostigmine 120 mg qid

4. clonidine 1mg hs

5. phenobarbital 1 gr bid

6. What is the interaction between Aricept and NSAID use?

7. Is it okay to take Depakote with the herbal evening primrose?

8. Is it okay to take Depakote with phenytoin?

9. Would a patient be on tizanidine and Avonex at the same time?

10. What is the black-box warning associated with pemoline?

PUZZLING THE TECHNICIAN

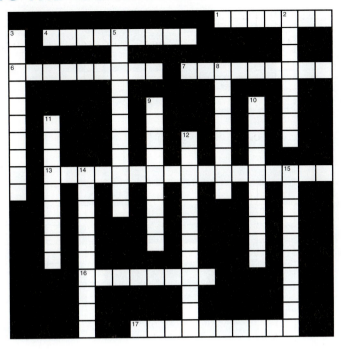

Across

1. brand name of the drug that is the dextro isomer of methylphenidate
4. first drug available in a class called catechol-o-methyl transferase
6. drug indicated for trauma-type seizures
7. drug that prevents metabolism of levodopa in the periphery
13. autoimmune disease where the patient gradually loses muscle function
16. drug that should not be taken with carbonated beverages
17. antiviral used to treat Parkinson's disease

Down

2. prodrug converted to dopamine
3. anticonvulsant that can cause kidney stones and weight loss
5. norepinephrine receptor blocker used to treat ADHD
8. only drug approved to treat amyotrophic lateral sclerosis
9. seizure where the patient has severe muscle jerks, but does not lose consciousness
10. tricyclic antidepressant found effective in attention-deficit hyperactivity disorder
11. prodrug converted to phenobarbital
12. prodrug converted to phenytoin
14. presence of these is characteristic of Parkinson's disease
15. MAOI found useful in Parkinson's disease

PUZZLING TERMINOLOGY

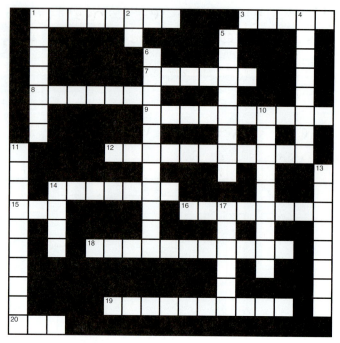

Across

1. another term for absence seizure
3. the part of a tablet that remains after the outer layer dissolves
7. a type of generalized seizure characterized by sudden loss of both muscle tone and consciousness
8. compounds that contain the same number and type of atoms but have exactly opposite (mirror image) structures
9. this disease is a degenerative disorder of the brain that leads to progressive dementia and changes in personality and behavior
12. involuntary contractions or series of contractions of the voluntary muscles
14. a type of generalized seizure characterized by a sudden, momentary break in consciousness; also called petit mal seizure
15. a neurologic disorder characterized by impulsivity and distractibility but with less hyperactivity than ADHD
16. the perception of two images of a single object
18. another term for grand mal seizure
19. this disease is a neurologic disorder characterized by akinesia, resting tremor, and muscular rigidity
20. a degenerative disease of the nerves; also called Lou Gehrig's disease

Down

1. this type of seizure is caused by an abnormal electrical discharge centered in a specific area of the brain; usually caused by a trauma
2. an autoimmune disease in which the myelin sheaths around nerves degenerate
4. abnormal electrical discharges in the cerebral cortex caused by sudden, excessive firing of neurons; result in a change in behavior of which the patient is not aware
5. a neurologic disorder of sudden and recurring seizures
6. symmetric, subcortical masses of gray matter embedded in the lower portions of the cerebral hemisphere; part of the extrapyramidal system; also called basal ganglia
10. a type of generalized seizure characterized by sudden muscle contractions with no loss of consciousness
11. imperfect articulation of speech
13. a type of generalized seizure characterized by body rigidity followed by muscle jerks; also called tonic-clonic seizure
14. a neurologic disorder characterized by hyperactivity, impulsivity, and distractibility
17. paralytic drooping of the upper eyelid

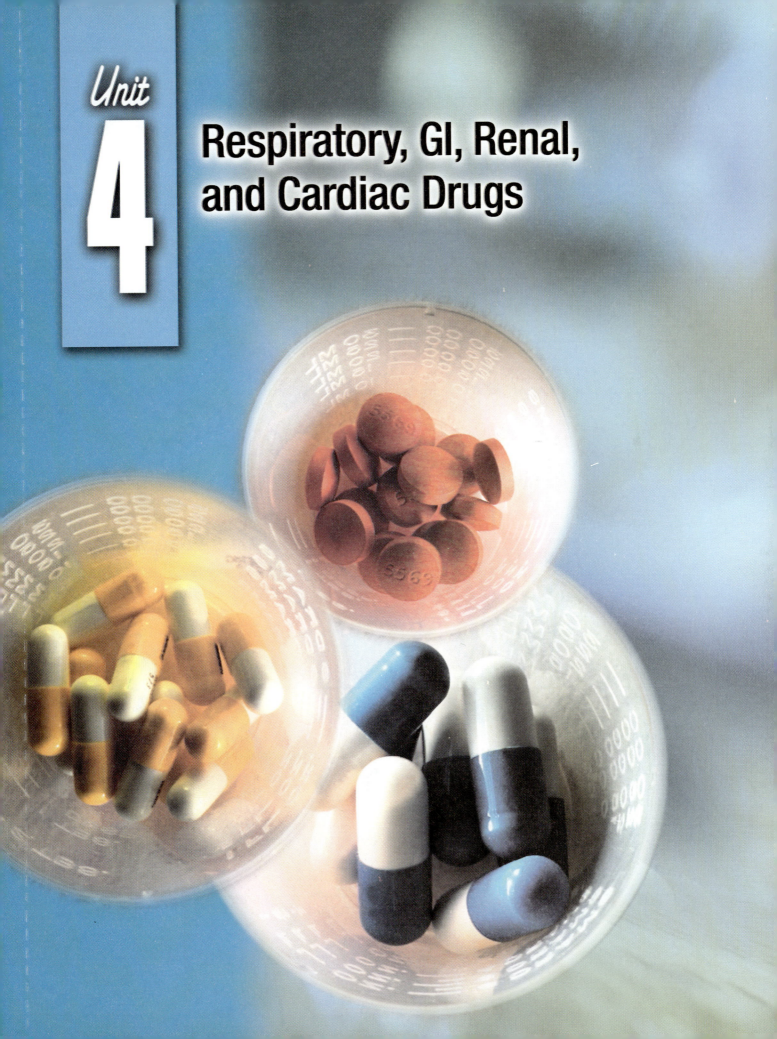
Unit 4
Respiratory, GI, Renal, and Cardiac Drugs

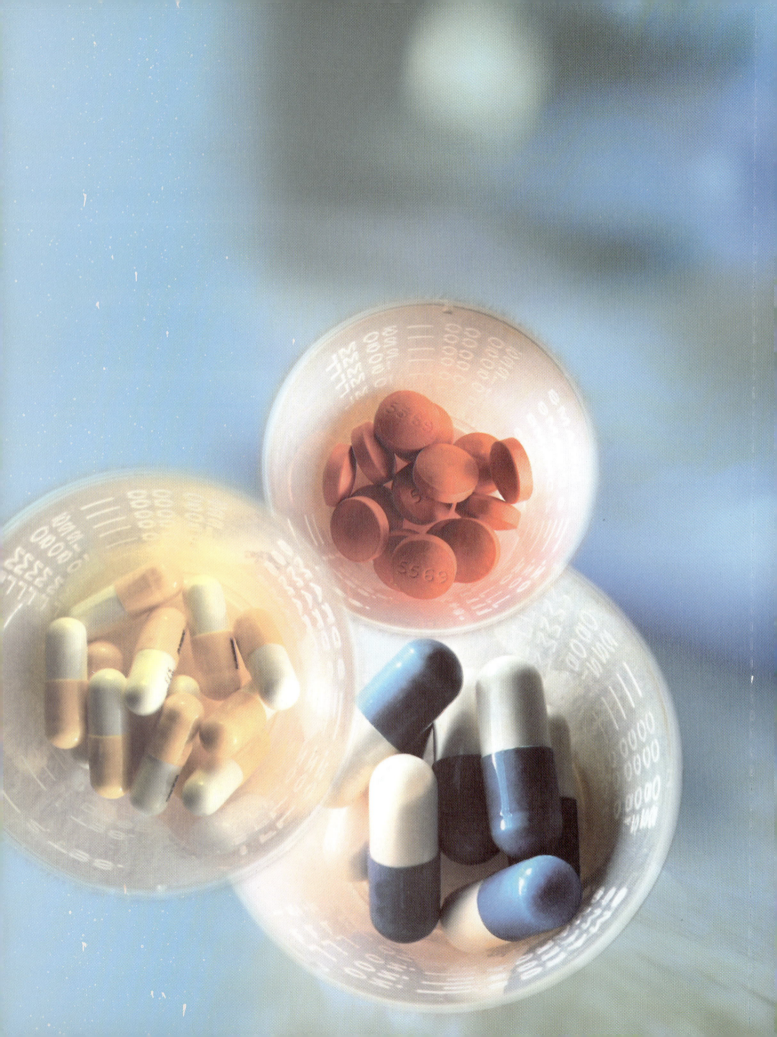

Respiratory Drugs

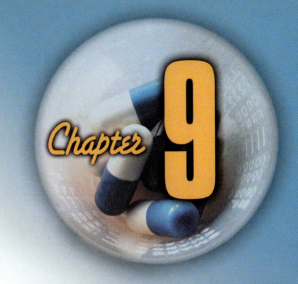

READING DRUG LABELS AND MEDICATION ORDERS

1. You receive the following prescription, and the label shown indicates the product to be dispensed. Based on the dosage prescribed, how long should the inhaler last?

   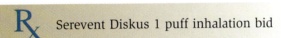

   Serevent Diskus 1 puff inhalation bid

   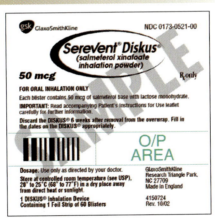

   For educational use only. Reproduced with permission of GlaxoSmithKline.

2. You receive the following prescription, and the product to be dispensed is available in a strenght of 100 mg/10 mg per 5 mL and the container is 120 mL.

   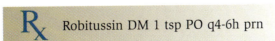

   Robitussin DM 1 tsp PO q4-6h prn

   a. How many bottles of this size would the patient need in order to get the maximum dosage for one week?

   b. Does the patient need a prescription to obtain this medication?

c. What are the active ingredients in this medication?
_____

3. Mr. Gaines brings in a prescription for the following cough syrup.

   ℞ Robitussin A-C 1 tsp PO q4-q6h prn persistent cough

   a. How would you express the directions on the label?
   _____
   _____

   b. What auxiliary labels would you add to this prescription bottle, and why?
   _____
   _____

   Guaifenesin Syrup and Dextrometh
   100 mg/10 mg per 5 mL
   120 mL

4. Mr. Marcos presents the following prescription to the pharmacy.

   ℞ Nicotine lozenge PO q4h prn cravings

   a. If Mr. Marcos uses the maximum number of lozenges every day, how many would he need for a month?
   _____

   b. What instructions should the patient receive about taking this medication?
   _____

5. A patient brings you the following prescription and the label indicates the product to be dispensed.

   ℞ Combivent 1 puff q4h-q6h prn

   a. By adding this new prescription, what two medications may be no longer required in the future?
   _____
   _____

   b. If the patient takes three puffs over the course of a day, how much of each drug would the patient receive in a day?
   _____
   _____
   _____

   NDC 0000-0000-00

   Ipratropium Bromide and Albuterol Sulfate

   200 metered doses
   14.7 g

   Each actuation delivers 18 mcg ipratropium bromide and 103 mcg albuterol sulfate from the mouthpiece.

   Caution: Federal law prohibits dispensing without prescription

6. You receive the following order in the pharmacy.

   ℞ Singulair 10 mg chew one tab PO daily

   a. Which dosage forms for Singulair are available to be given in this manner?
   _____

   b. How many tablets would you supply for one month?
   _____

7. You receive the following prescription in the pharmacy.

   ℞ Orapred 9 mg PO every day

   a. How large is the commercially available Orapred bottle?
   _____

   b. How long will this size bottle last this patient?
   _____

   c. How should this patient store Orapred?
   _____

8. You are working in an IV room in a hospital, and you receive the following order. The available stock label is also shown.

   ℞ Cipro 450 mg IV q12h

   NDC 0000-0000-00
   CIPROFLOXACIN
   Injection
   10 mg per mL
   40 mL
   Caution: Federal law prohibits dispensing without prescription

   a. If the stock solution shown in the drug label is provided, how many 400 mg vials would you use for a week of therapy?
   _____

   b. What is the closest dose of Cipro available in a premixed IV bag?
   _____

9. You receive the following prescription.

   ℞ rifampin 300 mg PO daily

   a. How many 150 mg capsules would the patient require for a three-month supply?
   _____

   b. If the patient required IV therapy, how would the dose change?
   _____

10. You receive the following prescription.

 Sudafed 60 mg PO 6h prn stuffiness

   a. Your pharmacy is currently out of Sudafed 60 mg tablets. What other tablet dosage forms are typically available to fill this prescription?
   _____

   b. How much of each dosage form would you require if the patient used Sudafed only three times a day?
   _____
   _____

11. You receive the following order.

 Vistaril 50 mg PO qhs

   a. Based on the prescription, which generic product would you dispense?
   _____

   b. What are the dosage forms available for this medication?
   _____

12. You receive the following prescription.

 Claritin 10 mg ng daily

   a. What dosage form would be appropriate for the nasogastric route?
   _____
   _____

   b. If the solution were preferred, and the solution is available as 1 mg/mL, how many teaspoonsful would be required per dose? (Note: 1 tsp = 5 mL. This and other equivalencies are available in the Pharmacy Library section of the IRC for this title at www.emcp.com.)
   _____

13. You receive the following prescription.

 beractant 4 mL/kg x 1 for RDS

   a. Detail how the preparation of this medication compares to Exosurf.
   _____

   b. Given the patient is 1.6 kg, how many 4 mL vials could the pharmacy be expected to dispense?
   _____

14. Unfortunately, Zyrtec-D is temporarily out of stock at the pharmacy. What could be a substitution if the following prescription is in the patient's profile?

> **Rx** Zyrtec-D 1 tab PO daily

_____
_____

UNDERSTANDING THE LARGER MEDICAL CONTEXT

1. You receive the following prescription. Which brand-name product would you expect to dispense and why?

    > **Rx** fluticasone 50 mcg, 1 spray daily

    _____

2. You receive the following set of prescriptions for a new asthma patient with mild, persistent asthma. What medication is most likely missing, and why is the missing medication important?

    > **Rx** Advair Diskus 250/50 inh bid

    > **Rx** Singulair 5 mg PO every day

    _____
    _____

3. Mrs. Banks comes into your pharmacy with symptoms consistent with allergic rhinitis. She has a history of uncontrolled hypertension. What OTC medications might she take for this condition?

    _____

4. Mr. Gates is a patient who has been coming in and out of your hospital for the past seven months. His most recent theophylline level was 6.8 mcg/mL, and he has been on theophylline 200 mg PO bid.

    a. What do you expect to happen to his dose?

    _____

    b. What factors could contribute to his level?

    _____
    _____

5. Mrs. Job, a pharmacy patient, has a severe reaction to peanuts.

   a. Which asthma medications should she avoid?
   _____

   b. What would be a long-acting alternative?
   _____

6. Ms. Bates presents the pharmacy with a list of medications that she takes on a regular basis.

   Atenolol 50 mg PO daily

   HCTZ 25 mg PO daily

   INH 300 mg PO daily

   a. What is the third drug on the list?
   _____

   b. Based on the dose of the third drug, which disease and phase is being treated.
   _____

7. Mr. Brightside has just been discharged from the hospital after being diagnosed with histoplasmosis. The physicians started him on oral antifungal therapy. He is also on a diet that requires him to eat one large meal at 4 pm every day.

   a. Which oral antifungal is Mr. Brightside most likely taking, and at what dose?
   _____

   b. Given the details of the patient's diet, how should he take his medication?
   _____
   _____

8. Mr. Usher takes the following regimen for his asthma.

   ℞ Advair 250/50 1 puff bid

   a. What should Mr. Usher do after taking his dose of Advair?
   _____

   b. How much fluticasone and salmeterol would Mr. Usher receive in one month? Show your calculation.
   _____
   _____

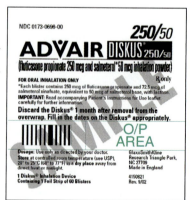

For educational use only. Reproduced with permission of GlaxoSmithKline.

c. Which two brand-name drugs does Advair Diskus replace?
_____

9. After another asthma attack, Mrs. Curry has been discharged from the hospital with a Medrol Dose Pack. Explain what a Medrol Dose Pack is, and detail how the methylprednisolone dosing depends on the day.
_____
_____

10. Ms. Lavigne has been a smoker for 35 years and has been diagnosed with asthma for 25 of those years. She is on lorazepam, which can cause respiratory depression. Because of a productive cough, she presents to your pharmacy with a request for her usual OTC cough syrup, although she cannot remember the name.

   a. What do you think her cough syrup may contain?
   _____
   _____

   b. List two brand-name medications that contain this active ingredient.
   _____

COMMUNICATING IN THE PHARMACY

1. Mrs. Dietz is a patient who uses your pharmacy. Her nephew will be living with her temporarily. She tells you that he has been diagnosed with cystic fibrosis; however, she does not know what the nephew's medications are.

   a. What uncommon medication used exclusively in cystic fibrosis should you make sure you have in stock?
   _____
   _____

   b. How does this medication work?
   _____
   _____

2. A medical student in the nursing home calls down to the pharmacy and asks, "Do you have Zantac 10 mg in stock? I don't see it in your formulary. Do you have Claritin in stock instead?"

   a. You suspect that the medical student has the wrong drug name. What medication might the student be looking for?
   _____

   b. What indication would make you think Zantac is not the intended drug?
   _____
   _____

3. While you are refilling the medications for the ER, a nurse asks if you are going to stock Xolair. She says, "My brother uses it, and I think I heard we can use it for asthma patients to stop attacks." What would the pharmacist tell her?

_____
_____
_____

4. You are training a new and inexperienced pharmacy technician. You receive the following prescription for a 59-year-old male. The technician gets the proper drug and fills the prescription. Before the pharmacist checks it, you notice there are no auxiliary labels on the packaging. What auxiliary labels would you suggest be added?

> ℞ Rifampin 300 mg PO daily

_____
_____
_____

DISPENSING AND STORING DRUGS

1. Where should dornase alfa be kept?
_____

2. What auxiliary labels would you place on a prescription for Robitussin A-C?
_____

3. Where should Spiriva capsules be kept?
_____

4. What three oral inhalers cannot be used in conjunction with a spacer?
_____

5. Where should the surfactants for respiratory distress syndrome be kept?
_____

6. You now have a new auxiliary label entitled "For acute use in case of asthma attack." Which medications could use this label?
_____

7. What auxiliary label is found on vials of Tessalon Pearls, Zyban, and Nicoderm lozenges?
_____

8. What auxiliary label is placed on a Benadryl prescription?

9. Which auxiliary label would you include on a bottle of Lugol solution?

10. Which medication should receive an auxiliary label that reads "Do not use for more that three consecutive days"?

PUTTING SAFETY FIRST

Does the requested dose match the typical medication dose in the following orders? If not, provide the typical dosage for each medication.

1. Spiriva 1 tab PO daily

2. theophylline 300 mg cap PO q12h

3. benzonatate 100 mg PO q12h

4. Antivert 125 mg PO q6h prn vertigo symptoms

5. diphenhydramine 50 mg PO ac qam

6. buproprion 75 mg PO qid for nicotine dependence

7. Survanta 5 mL PO q4h prn tracheal dryness

8. Nasalcrom 2 puff qid prn

9. Nasonex 50 mcg spray every day

10. Advair Diskus 50 mcg inh bid

PUZZLING THE TECHNICIAN

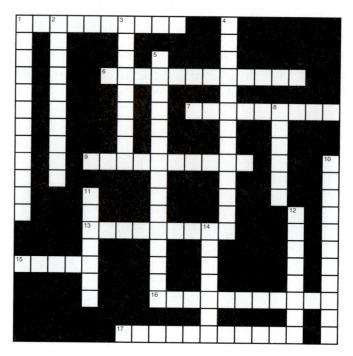

Across

1. first antihistamine nasal spray, generic name
6. xanthine derivative that has a therapeutic blood level range of 10 mcg/mL to 20 mcg/mL, generic name
7. generic name for RDS drug derived from cattle lung
9. monoclonal antibody for asthma, generic name
13. brand name for dornase alfa
15. antidepressant also used for nicotine dependence treatment, brand name
16. subcutaneous drug for *status asthmaticus*
17. generic name for Vistaril

Down

1. preferred IV therapy for histoplasmosis
2. brand name for budesonide product not used for asthma treatment
3. medical term that means "fast breathing"
4. generic name for Clarinex
5. chemical name for Lugol solution
8. least-sedating OTC antihistamine, brand name
10. Singulair, Zyflo, and Accolate are all examples of ____ inhibitors
11. S isomer for albuterol, brand name
12. major metabolite of nicotine
14. brand name for guaifenesin tablets

PUZZLING TERMINOLOGY

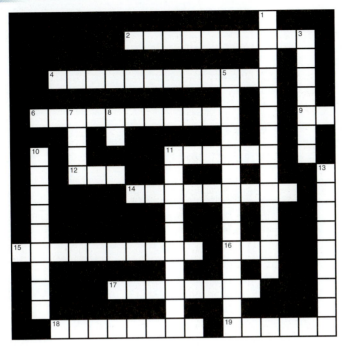

Across

2. agents that destroy or dissolve mucus
4. an agent that causes the mucous membranes to shrink, thereby allowing the sinus cavities to drain
6. an agent that decreases the thickness and stickiness of mucus, enabling the patient to rid the lungs and airway of mucus when coughing
9. a disease of the lungs and other body tissues and organs caused by Mycobacterium tuberculosis
11. a reversible lung disease with intermittent attacks in which inspiration is obstructed; provoked by airborne allergens
12. a syndrome occurring in newborns that is characterized by acute asphyxia with hypoxia and acidosis
14. an irreversible lung disease characterized by destruction of the alveoli in the lungs, which allows air to accumulate in tissues and organs
15. an antibody produced in a laboratory from an isolated specific lymphocyte that produces a pure antibody against a known specific antigen
16. a device that delivers a specific amount of medication in a puff of compressed gas
17. a major metabolite of nicotine
18. receptors in the lungs and airways that respond to coarse particles and chemicals, causing a cough
19. a device used with a MDI to decrease the amount of spray deposited on the back of the throat and swallowed

Down

1. a respiratory tract infection caused by a fungus, most often found in accumulated droppings from birds and bats; often called the summer flu
3. receptors in the lungs and airways that respond to elongation of muscle, causing a cough
5. common term for drugs that block the H1 receptors
7. the maximum flow rate generated during a forced expiration, measured in liters per minute
8. a hereditary disorder of infants, children, and young adults that involves widespread dysfunction of the gastrointestinal and pulmonary systems
10. a common lung infection, caused by microorganisms that gain access to the lower respiratory tract
11. inhalation of fluids from the mouth and throat
13. a device used in the administration of inhaled medications; uses air flowing past a liquid to create a mist

Gastrointestinal Drugs and Related Diseases

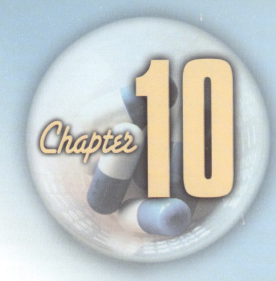

Chapter 10

READING DRUG LABELS AND MEDICATION ORDERS

1. A patient comes into your pharmacy with the following prescription. If the patient took this medication as frequently as the prescription allows, how long would it take for a pint-sized bottle to run out?

    Maalox 1 tbsp PO tid prn heartburn

   _____

   _____

2. A patient comes into your pharmacy with a prescription stating "Prevpac, use as directed." The drug label shown is the product you pick up from the pharmacy shelf.

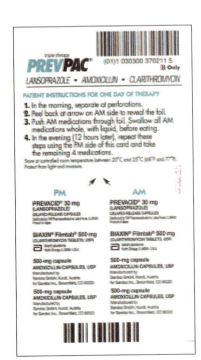

Courtesy of TAP Pharmaceuticals Inc., Lake Forest, IL. Used with permission.

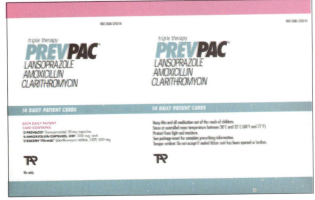

Name _____ Date _____

a. What are the individual drugs in this product, and what are their respective dosage forms and dosage strengths?

_____

_____

b. How many total pills will be taken per day?

_____

3. Mr. Bryk is 26 years old, 172 lb, and 5'7". Because he has Crohn's disease, he is starting Remicade. The drug label shown indicates the product he is going to be taking. During his induction period, his dose will be 5 mg/kg. (*Note:* 1 kg = 2.2 lb. This and other equivalencies are available in the Pharmacy Library section of the IRC for this title at www.emcp.com.)

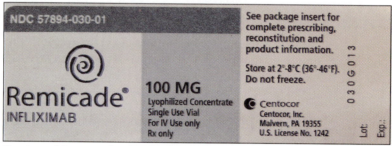

Courtesy of Centocor, Inc. Used with permission.

a. How many total milligrams will he require per dose during the induction period?

_____

b. How many vials will he require per dose during the induction period?

_____

c. What would you choose as a final solution volume if the usual concentration for Remicade is 1–2 mg/mL?

_____

_____

4. Mr. Griffiths has been diagnosed with recurrent gallstones. He is currently using Actigall at prophylaxis doses. His doctor has written the following prescription. Based on the smallest available capsule size for this medication, how many capsules will Mr. Griffiths receive in a month?

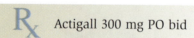 Actigall 300 mg PO bid

_____

5. Mr. Sim has been given a prescription for Enulose, and the following drug label shows the product available in the pharmacy.

 Enulose 2 tbsp PO q6h prn constipation

a. How many grams of lactulose will Mr. Sim be getting in a dose?

b. How many doses will Mr. Sim be able to get from a bottle of Enulose, assuming no waste?

c. How many days of treatment will a bottle last if Mr. Sim takes the maximum dosage per day?

16 Fl Oz (473 mL)
NDC 0000-0000-00

Lactulose Syrup USP
10 g/15 mL

FOR ORAL OR RECTAL ADMINISTRATION

Each 15 mL of syrup contains 10 g lactulose

Caution: Federal law prohibits dispensing without prescription

6. Mr. Lazar is on mesalamine 800 mg PO tid.

   a. Which brand-name product should Mr. Lazar receive?

   b. What will be the directions on the medication label?

7. Mr. Hepp has been instructed to take Pepto-Bismol for his traveler's diarrhea. What is the generic name for Pepto-Bismol?

8. Mrs. Tollan has started on GoLYTELY before her colonoscopy tomorrow.

   a. How many milliliters should Mrs. Tollan add to the jug to prepare the dose?

   b. How many 8 fl oz doses are in the 4 L jug?

9. Miss Anderson, a Hepatitis C positive patient, brings the following prescription to your pharmacy.

   ℞ Copegus 600 mg PO bid

   a. If the tablets are 200 mg, how many tablets will she receive in one day?

   b. What other medication should accompany the Copegus? Why?

10. Mr. Doole requires ranitidine in his total parenteral nutrition (TPN) for stress ulcer prophylaxis. The recommended dose is 150 mg/day. How many milliliters of Zantac for injection would Mr. Doole get in each TPN?

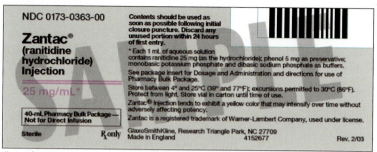

For educational use only. Reproduced with permission of GlaxoSmithKline.

UNDERSTANDING THE LARGER MEDICAL CONTEXT

1. Mr. Whitney has been HIV-positive for four years. His medication regimen during that time period has included Lipitor 20 mg PO daily, Toprol-XL 100 mg PO daily, albuterol inhaler 1–2 puffs qid prn wheezing, Sustiva 600 mg PO daily, and Combivir 1 tab bid. Unfortunately, he now is diagnosed as having active hepatitis B. Which of these medications would you predict his HBV will be resistant to? Why?

2. Mrs. Copeland is 28 years old, 168 cm tall, and 170 lb. Would she qualify for Xenical therapy? Why or why not?

3. What medication might be prescribed to a patient with leg cramps and malaria?

4. To increase the chances for successful treatment of hepatitis C, which medication must be used with Copegus?

5. What medication might benefit a patient with nausea secondary to gastroparesis?

6. Which medication can treat both diarrhea and constipation?

7. Which combination medication has ingredients that could cause both diarrhea and constipation if the generic components were used separately in high doses?

8. What is the class prototype for stool softeners?

9. Which class of antiemetics is most effective for treatment of emesis in highly emetogenic chemotherapy?

10. Give two examples of medications from the above class (question 9).

COMMUNICATING IN THE PHARMACY

1. You have a new technician who is four months pregnant. Which gastrointestinal system medication that prevents stomach ulcers should she avoid handling?

2. A nurse calls the pharmacy looking for a missing diarrhea medication. Which medications of this class are controlled substances?

3. What additional precautions should be taken within the pharmacy when filling a medication order for azathioprine?

4. Mr. Johnson comes to the pharmacy window for a refill of Dulcolax. What would you do?

5. Mrs. Clarkson comes to your pharmacy in the late afternoon because she has been having GERD symptoms. She asks you where the Prilosec OTC is. You show her where it is on the shelves, and the last thing she says to you is, "Thank you. I am happy that I'll feel better tonight before bed." What should you do?

DISPENSING AND STORING DRUGS

Where should the following medications be stored in the pharmacy?

1. Pepcid IV

2. Pegasys

3. loperamide solution

4. amoxicillin suspension after reconstitution

5. Remicade IV

6. Carafate suspension

7. Protonix IV

8. Intron A

9. Epivir-HBV

What auxiliary labels would you put on the following medications?
10. primaquine tablet

11. metronidazole

12. Bactrim suspension

13. praziquantel tablets

14. Mr. Bacon has had diarrhea for the past three days due to a change in diet. His physician has started him on loperamide 4 mg PO q4h prn loose stool.

   a. What is the maximum dose of loperamide for one day of therapy?

   b. What will the medication label say about the maximum dosage?

PUTTING SAFETY FIRST

Do the doses match the medications? If not, give a common dose.

1. Prilosec 30 mg PO daily
   _____

2. Zantac 20 mg PO daily
   _____

3. Kytril 24 mg 30 minutes before chemotherapy
   _____

4. Asacol 800 mg PO tid
   _____

5. Zelnorm 60 mg PO bid
   _____

If there is a potential interaction between these drug pairs, identify it.

6. Protonix and Reyataz
   _____

7. Maalox and Levaquin
   _____

8. paregoric and lorazepam
   _____

9. psyllium and digoxin
   _____

PUZZLING THE TECHNICIAN

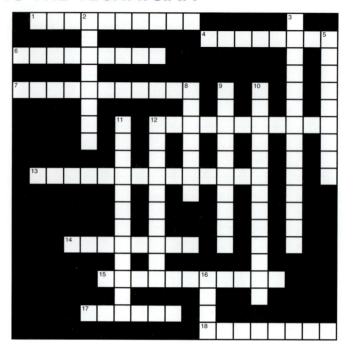

Across

1. active ingredient for Asacol, Pentasa, and Rowasa
4. brand name for meclizine
6. brand name for promethazine
7. pink suspension helpful in treating traveler's diarrhea, brand name
12. silicon polymer
13. topical steroid for hemorrhoids
14. brand name for ursodiol
15. generic name for Aciphex
17. word for vomiting
18. stool softener

Down

2. generic for Hepsera
3. antiemetic that promotes GI motility
5. 5-HT$_4$ agonist
8. brand name for diphenoxylate-atropine
9. oral steroid for Crohn's disease
10. antiparasitic that inhibits ATP synthesis
11. generic for Creon-10, Viokase, and Pancrease
12. agent that protects ulcers by forming a protective coat over the ulceration
16. brand name for nizatidine

PUZZLING TERMINOLOGY

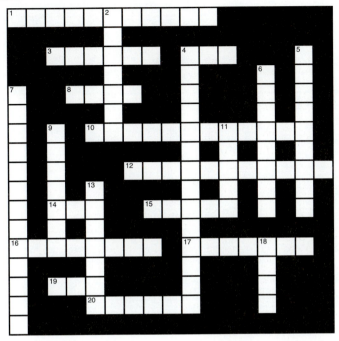

Across

1. drugs that inhibit impulses that cause vomiting from going to the stomach
3. backflow; specifically in GERD, the backflow of acidic stomach contents across an incompetent lower esophageal sphincter
4. an area below the floor of the fourth ventricle of the brain that can trigger nausea and vomiting when certain signals are received
8. a GI disease characterized by radiating burning or pain in the chest and an acid taste, caused by backflow of acidic stomach contents across an incompetent lower esophageal sphincter; also called heartburn
10. a local excavation in the gastric mucosa
12. stool softeners that have a detergent activity that facilitates admixture of fat and water to make the stool soft and mushy
14. a functional disorder in which the lower GI tract does not have appropriate tone or spasticity to regulate bowel activity
15. the undigested residue of fruits, vegetables, and other foods of plant origin that remains after digestion by the human GI enzymes
16. single-cell organisms that inhabit water and soil
17. a state in which an individual's total body weight includes greater quantities of fat than is considered normal (25% of total body weight for men and 35% for women)
19. a guide to use in determining whether to initiate pharmacologic treatment for obesity; calculated by dividing patient's weight (in kilograms) by patient's height (in meters) squared
20. an inflammatory bowel disease affecting the entire GI tract from mouth to anus

Down

2. an infectious febrile disease transmitted by the anopheles mosquito
4. a GI and pulmonary disease; GI effects involve increased viscosity of mucous secretions and relative deficiencies of pancreatic enzymes
5. irritation and superficial erosion of the stomach lining
6. an agent that stimulates bowel content removal by increasing osmolarity of bowel fluids
7. impaired intestinal absorption of nutrients
9. the sensation of the room spinning when one gets up or changes positions; can be treated with anticholinergic agents
11. a local defect or excavation of the surface of an organ or tissue
13. laxatives (stool softeners) that draw water into the colon and thereby stimulate evacuation
18. the notation for immune globulin that is given intravenously

Urinary System Drugs

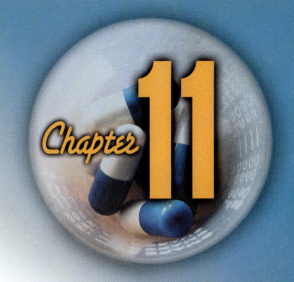

Chapter 11

READING DRUG LABELS AND MEDICATION ORDERS

1. You receive the following prescription, and the product available in the pharmacy is 5 mg/mL of oral liquid in a 473 mL container.

   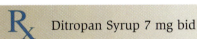 Ditropan Syrup 7 mg bid

   a. How much do you need to dispense for a 30-day supply?
   _____

   b. If you dispensed the entire bottle, how long would it last the patient?
   _____

2. You receive the following prescription, and the drug label shown is the product available in the pharmacy. Can you fill this prescription with the drug shown? Why or why not?

   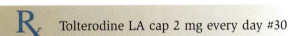 Tolterodine LA cap 2 mg every day #30

   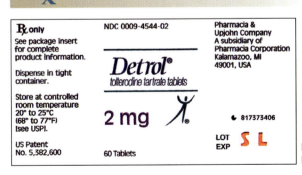

   Reproduced with permission of Pfizer Inc. All rights reserved.

   _____
   _____
   _____

3. You receive the following prescription, and the drug label shown is the product available in the pharmacy.

℞ Lupron Depot 3 as directed

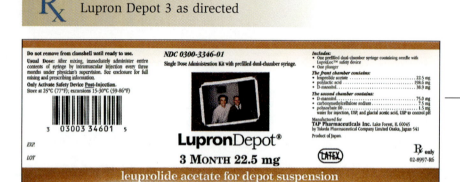

Courtesy of TAP Pharmaceuticals Inc., Lake Forest, IL. Used with permission.

a. Is this the correct product? If not, why not?

b. How will this be administered?

c. How long will this dose last?

4. You receive the following prescription, and the product available in the pharmacy is available as 40 mg/mL in a 240 mL container.

℞ Megace Susp 60 mg bid

a. How long will this bottle last the patient?

b. Is it okay to also fill a prescription for metronidazole for this patient? If not, why not?

5. You receive the following prescription.

℞ Torsemide 20 mg IV every day

a. The pharmacy has a 2 mL and a 5 mL size of 10 mg/mL. Which of the two products do you choose to fill the prescription? Why?

_____

_____

b. When added to D_5W, how long is the solution stable at room temperature?

_____

UNDERSTANDING THE LARGER MEDICAL CONTEXT

1. Which bacteria causes most urinary tract infections?

_____

_____

2. What are the common side effects of a potassium-sparing diuretic?

_____

_____

_____

3. What are the stages of renal disease?

_____

_____

_____

_____

4. Which classes of diuretics require potassium supplementation, and which ones do not?

_____

_____

5. What are the symptoms of chronic renal insufficiency?

_____

_____

_____

_____

6. Why should tricyclic antidepressants be avoided in patients with BPH?

_____

_____

_____

_____

7. Why is antibiotic treatment for UTIs usually limited to three days instead of the seven to 10 days used for other infections?

   _____
   _____
   _____
   _____

8. How does kidney failure cause anemia?

   _____
   _____

9. What are the benefits of switching from Ditropan XL to Oxytrol?

   _____
   _____
   _____

10. What role does testosterone play in BPH?

    _____
    _____
    _____

COMMUNICATING IN THE PHARMACY

1. Mr. Brown brings in his new prescription for furosemide. The directions are for dosing twice a day. What should you tell Mr. Brown about taking this new drug?

   _____
   _____
   _____
   _____

2. Mr. Long brings his new prescription for doxazosin into your pharmacy. He wants to know if you can fill it for him. He currently is on furosemide, amlodipine, and metoprolol from a different physician. Do you fill this prescription today? Why or why not?

   _____
   _____
   _____
   _____

3. A nurse calls down from one of the floors and asks you if a patient can be on furosemide and metolazone at the same time. What information should be relayed to the nurse?

___

4. While Mrs. Verzi is waiting for her prescription for oxybutynin to be refilled, she asks you to recommend a stool softener. She mentions being constipated the last couple of weeks. What can you tell Mrs. Verzi?

___

5. A patient is complaining about the cost of her prescription for Ferrex 150 Forte (polysaccharide-iron complex with vitamin B) at your pharmacy. She wants to know why it is worth more than the cheaper iron available.

___

DISPENSING AND STORING DRUGS

What auxiliary labels would you put on the following medications?
1. ferrous sulfate

   ___

2. Bactrim DS

   ___

3. doxazosin

   ___

4. metolazone

   ___

5. ciprofloxacin

   ___

Name ___ Date ___

6. hydrochlorothiazide

7. Oxytrol

8. nitrofurantoin

9. Uroxatral

10. Aranesp

Where would you find the following medications in a pharmacy?

11. phenazopyridine

12. Epogen

13. CellCept

14. Nephrocaps is a brand of vitamins specially formulated for dialysis patients. What is in Nephrocaps?

PUTTING SAFETY FIRST

Does the requested dose match the typical medication dose in the following orders? If not, provide the typical dosage for each medication.

1. metolazone 10 mg bid

2. bethanechol 25 mg tid

3. Cipro 500 mg bid x 10 days for uncomplicated UTI

4. finasteride 1 mg daily for BPH

5. HCTZ 50 mg daily
   _____

6. Oxytrol apply 1 patch every other day
   _____

7. Aranesp 25 mcg SC every 12 days
   _____

8. furosemide 20 mg TID
   _____

9. Why is it important to take iron supplements at a time different from that of other medications?
   _____
   _____
   _____

Name _____ Date _____

PUZZLING THE TECHNICIAN

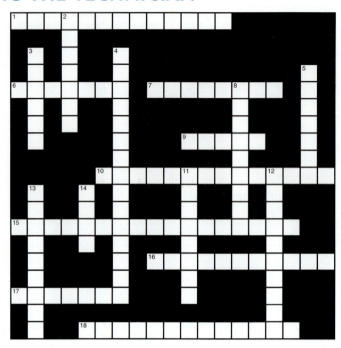

Across

1. immunosuppressant used for kidney transplants
6. time of day recommended for patients to take alpha-1 receptor blockers
7. procedure used to filter the blood in patients with kidney failure
9. brand name for bumetanide
10. diuretic that can cause gynecomastia in males
15. inhibitor class of drug that acetazolamide is in
16. penicillin antibiotic that is dosed tid for UTI
17. brand-name drug that combines a potassium-sparing and non-potassium-sparing diuretic
18. amino acid reduced by dialysis

Down

2. category of diuretics of mannitol
3. syndrome where excess urea is maintained in the blood
4. OTC urinary tract anesthetic that will turn urine orange
5. brand name of the drug for interstitial cystitis
8. drug used for hyperphosphatemia
11. units that produce urine in the kidneys
12. alpha-1 receptor blocker that is highly selective for prostate tissue; little effect on blood pressure
13. drug that increases bladder volume by reducing spasticity of the detrussor muscle
14. class of diuretics that works at the loop of Henle

PUZZLING TERMINOLOGY

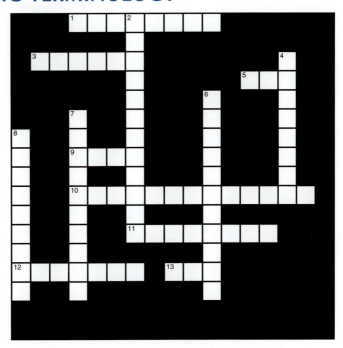

Across

1. a substance that rids the body of excess fluid and electrolytes by increasing the urine output
3. the clinical syndrome resulting from renal dysfunction in which excessive products of protein metabolism are retained in the blood
5. abnormal enlargement of the prostate gland, usually associated with aging
9. diuretics that inhibit reabsorption of sodium and chloride in the loop of Henle, thereby causing increased urinary output
10. immature red blood cells
11. glomerulotubular units that are the working units of the kidney
12. diuretics that increase the osmotic pressure of glomerular filtrate, thereby inhibiting tubular reabsorption of water and electrolytes and increasing urinary output
13. infection caused by bacteria, usually *E. coli*, that enter via the urethra and progress up the urinary tract

Down

2. the process by which substances are pulled back into the blood after waste products have been removed during the formation of urine
4. diuretics that promote sodium and water excretion in the urine, lower the sodium level in vessel walls, and reduce vasoconstriction
6. the proportion of red blood cells to the total volume of blood
7. the removal of substances from the blood as part of the formation of urine by the renal tubules
8. the release of cell products, including hydrogen and potassium ions and acids and bases, during urine formation

Cardiovascular Drugs

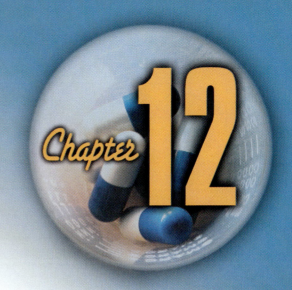

READING DRUG LABELS AND MEDICATION ORDERS

1. You receive the following prescription, and the drug label shown is the product you pick up from the pharmacy shelf.

    Catapres patch 0.2 mg q7d

   a. How many 0.2 mg patches will the patient receive for a month's supply?

   _____

   _____

   b. A box of Catapres has been opened, and you want to confirm that no contents have been removed. What comes in a box of Catapres?

   _____

   NDC 0000-0000-00 — Transdermal use only

   CLONIDINE

   Transdermal Therapeutic System

   4 patches and 4 adhesive covers

   Delivery of 0.2 mg clonidine per day for one week.

   Caution: Federal law prohibits dispensing without prescription

2. You receive the following prescription, and the available drug contains 4 g of resin in 9 g of powder.

    cholestyramine 1 packet PO tid

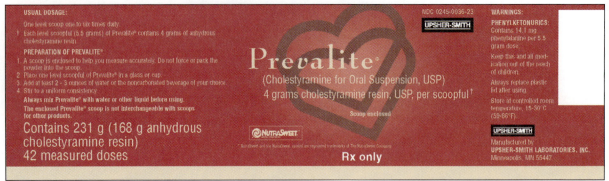

Reprinted with permission of Upsher-Smith. All rights reserved.

    a. How many grams would the patient receive in one day?

    _____

    b. How should this product be prepared before administration?

    _____

3. You receive the following order, and the drug label shown is the product you pick up from the pharmacy shelf.

 Amiodarone 900 mg/500 mg IV per atrial arrhythmia protocol

    a. How many milliliters of amiodarone would you require to make this product?

    _____

    b. Why must a filter be used when administering intravenous amiodarone?

    _____
    _____

4. You receive the following order.

 Metoprolol 400 mg PO daily

    a. What is the brand name for the product you will dispense?

    _____

    b. What is the largest tablet that you could possibly use to fill the prescription, and how many of these tablets would be required for a month's supply?

    _____
    _____

5. You receive the following prescription.

   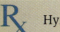 Hyzaar 50/12.5 1 tab PO daily

   a. What are the generic ingredients in this product?
   _____

   b. How many milligrams of diuretic will the patient receive in one month?
   _____

6. You receive the following order for Mr. Brosnan. He is a 65-year-old man with a history of pulmonary hypertension. The patient's weight is 87 kg, and the patient's home dose is prepared in a 30,000 ng/mL, 100 mL CADD pump cassette.

    Flolan 16 ng/kg/min

   a. Since the patient must receive that concentration, how many 1.5 mg vials should you use to prepare it? Show your calculation.
   _____

   b. How many milliliters will the patient receive in one day of therapy? Show your calculation.
   _____
   _____

7. You receive the following prescription, and the drug is available as a 20 mg/mL injection.

    hydralazine 20 mg IV q6h

   a. The hospital requires a five-day supply to be stored in an automated dispensing machine on the floor. How many vials would you send to the floor?
   _____

   b. If the dose were reduced to 10 mg IV q6h, how would the number of vials sent to the floor change?
   _____

8. You receive the following prescription.

    Lovenox (enoxaparin) 90 mg SC bid

a. Which product would you select to fill this prescription?

b. How many milliliters would correspond to the 90 mg dose?

9. You receive the following prescription.

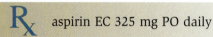
aspirin EC 325 mg PO daily

a. What does EC stand for?

b. How would this differ from a prescription for baby aspirin?

10. You are assembling some pharmacy kits for the intensive care units at your hospital. The kit contains

   #1 125 mg vial of diltiazem for injection

   #1 100 mL bag of sodium chloride

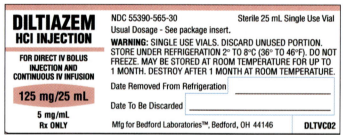
Used with permission of Bedford Laboratories.

a. If these two products were added together, what would the resultant concentration be?

b. Where would this kit be stored?

UNDERSTANDING THE LARGER MEDICAL CONTEXT

1. You are filling the medication cassettes at your hospital, and you notice that both a Catapres 0.2 mg patch and clonidine 0.1 mg tablets have been ordered for a patient in the ICU. Under what circumstances might these medications be used together?

2. While performing a medication delivery, you are told that the same patient in the ICU has been on nitroglycerin, dopamine, and nitroprusside drips continuously for 72 hours. The nurse tells you that she needs twice as much of all three items stocked because of the high rate. Why do you relay this information back to the pharmacist?

_____
_____

3. Mr. Harris is a patient of your pharmacy who has recently been diagnosed with hyperlipidemia. His physician has him on Lipitor 20 mg PO daily. In addition to drug therapy, what lifestyle changes could Mr. Harris make to decrease his risks for cardiovascular disease?

_____
_____

4. Mr. Banks walks into your pharmacy. He asks you to get him some Tylenol and Emetrol because he has been feeling nauseous and having headaches. As you ring him out, he mutters that everything looks yellow and out of focus. What drug reaction might this patient be experiencing?

_____
_____

5. Mrs. Miller is a type I diabetic with a history of hypertension for 13 years. Her physician attempted to start her on lisinopril 10 mg PO daily; however, she developed angioedema and will not rechallenge the reaction. If her physician still wants to control her hypertension by affecting angiotensin, which medications might the physician prescribe?

_____
_____

6. In general, why are decongestants contraindicated in patients with cardiovascular disease?

_____
_____

COMMUNICATING IN THE PHARMACY

1. A hospital patient is taking Natrecor. The patient's nurse calls you because she will run out of the medication in 10 minutes and does not have another bag to hang in its place. You notice that you have a bag for the patient that will go up on the next run in 30 minutes. She asks you to use the hospital pneumatic tube system to get it to her sooner. What do you tell her?

_____
_____

2. Mr. Jarkko was discharged from City Hospital after recovery from a stroke he had while taking Plavix. His physician has started him on Aggrenox. As you

begin to ring up his prescription, along with a bottle of aspirin and several other items, he looks at the patient information sheet and says, "I didn't know this had aspirin in it. You can delete that from my order." You alert the pharmacist. What do you expect the pharmacist will explain to the patient about this medication?

_____

_____

3. A nurse calls from the floor and asks for another Covera HS tablet, because she gave the medication at the beginning of her shift and the patient's blood pressure is still 195/110. What would you ask her before sending another dose?

_____

_____

4. Mr. West comes in to pick up his prescription for Lotensin, and he mentions he has had a cough. You ask him to describe the cough. He calls it a dry cough, but he has been feeling fine otherwise. What would you do?

_____

_____

5. You are delivering medications to the hospital floors when you hear a commotion. The nurse tells you that a bag of heparin accidentally ran at four times the rate, and the patient is starting to bleed. Immediately you pick up the phone to call the pharmacy. A newly trained technician answers. What medication will you ask the technician to get from the pharmacist, because the patient will require it soon? Why?

_____

_____

DISPENSING AND STORING DRUGS

How should the following medications be stored in the pharmacy?

1. eptifibatide injection

    _____

2. NTG tablets after opening

    _____

3. Isuprel ampules

    _____

4. atropine vials

    _____

5. nitroprusside injection

    _____

6. alteplase before and after reconstitution
   _____

7. Flolan cassette
   _____

8. digoxin tablets
   _____

9. Lovenox syringes
   _____

10. Cardura tablets
    _____

What auxiliary labels would you put on the following medications?

11. Lipitor tablets
    _____

12. nifedipine XL
    _____

13. antihypertensives
    _____

14. TriCor
    _____

15. Questran and WelChol
    _____

PUTTING SAFETY FIRST

Does the dose match the medication? If not, give a common dose.

1. propafenone 50 mg PO bid
   _____

2. terazosin 2 mg PO qam
   _____

3. clonidine patch 0.2 mg apply daily
   _____

4. Imdur 0.4 mg PO q5min prn chest pain, repeat up to 3 times
   _____

5. Natrecor 1.5 mg PO daily
   _____

6. hydralazine 50 mg PO qhs

7. Lovenox 5 mg PO daily

8. Lipitor 40 mg PO daily

9. Zetia 100 mg PO daily

10. Cardizem CD 240 mg PO bid

11. Lanoxin 125 mg PO daily

12. Lopressor 150 mg PO daily

13. Procardia XL 90 mg ng daily

14. Avapro 750 mg PO daily

15. guanfacine 1 mg PO tid

PUZZLING THE TECHNICIAN

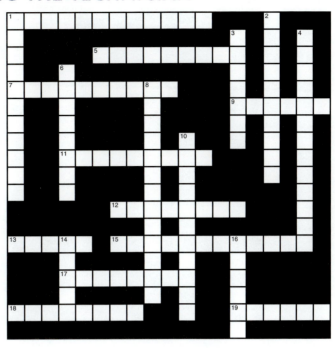

Across

1. antidote for warfarin overdose
5. when used in high doses, this local anesthetic has antiarrythmic properties
7. class III antiarrythmic that is available IV and PO
9. monoclonal antibody sometimes used for clot prevention during angioplasty; brand name
11. most potent alpha blocker
12. antihyperlipidemic present in your diet; similar to Niaspan
13. blocks absorption of cholesterol in the small intestine
15. drug for pulmonary hypertension; infused by a subcutaneous pump
17. antidote for Lanoxin overdose
18. combination product containing aspirin and dipyridamole
19. 100 times more specific for aldosterone than spironolactone

Down

1. generic name for Rythmol
2. one of two generics contained in combination drug Zestoretic
3. drug titrated according to PTT results
4. used for atropine-resistant bradyarrythmias
6. inhibits clotting factors II, VII, IX, X and is monitored by INR measurement
8. when given by transdermal route, this medication must be taken off for eight hours
10. generic for Angiomax
14. brand name for the isosorbide-containing nitrate that is dosed once a day
16. least common of all drugs used to prevent stroke, due to agranulocytosis

PUZZLING TERMINOLOGY

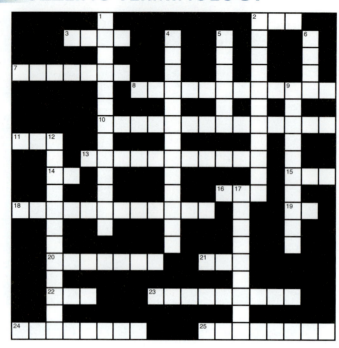

Across

2. a condition in which the heart can no longer pump adequate blood to the body's tissues; results in engorgement of the pulmonary vessels
3. neurologic changes that reverse spontaneously but less rapidly than a TIA
7. a pacemaker other than the SA node
8. enlargement of the heart due to overwork from overstimulation
10. spasmodic or suffocating chest pain caused by an imbalance between oxygen supply and oxygen demand
11. a lipoprotein containing 5% triglyceride, 25% cholesterol, and 50% protein; "good cholesterol"
13. a Class II antiarrhythmic drug that competitively blocks response to beta stimulation; decreases heart rate, myocardial contractility, blood pressure, and myocardial oxygen demand; used to treat arrhythmias, MIs, and angina
14. sudden blocking of the pulmonary artery by a blood clot
15. temporary neurologic changes that occur over a brief period of time; may be a warning sign and predictor of imminent stroke
16. lipoprotein containing 6% triglycerides and 65% cholesterol; "bad cholesterol"
18. elevated blood pressure, where systolic blood pressure is greater than 140 mm Hg and diastolic pressure is greater than 90 mm Hg
19. a heart attack; occurs when a region of the heart muscle is deprived of oxygen
20. stationary blood clots
21. a test that measures the function of the intrinsic and common pathways; affected by heparin
22. a method of standardizing the prothrombin time (PT) by comparing it to a standard index
23. arterial impedance, or the force against which cardiac muscle shortens; along with preload and contractility, determines cardiac output
24. a blood pressure measurement that measures the pressure during contraction of the heart
25. stroke resulting from cerebral infarction, in which a region of the brain is deprived of oxygen

Down

1. a class of drugs that reduce the risk of clot formation by inhibiting platelet aggregation
2. an odorless, white, waxlike, powdery substance that is present in all foods of animal origin but not in foods of plant origin; circulates continuously in the blood for use by all body cells
4. a class of agents that dissolve clots
5. the result of an event (finite, ongoing, or protracted occurrences) that interrupts oxygen supply to an area of the brain; usually caused by cerebral infarction or cerebral hemorrhage
6. lipoprotein containing 60% triglycerides and 12% cholesterol
9. any variation from the normal heartbeat
12. spherical particles containing a core of triglycerides and cholesterol, in varying proportions, surrounded by a surface coat of phospholipids so that they can remain in solution
17. the blood pressure measurement that measures the pressure during the dilation of the heart

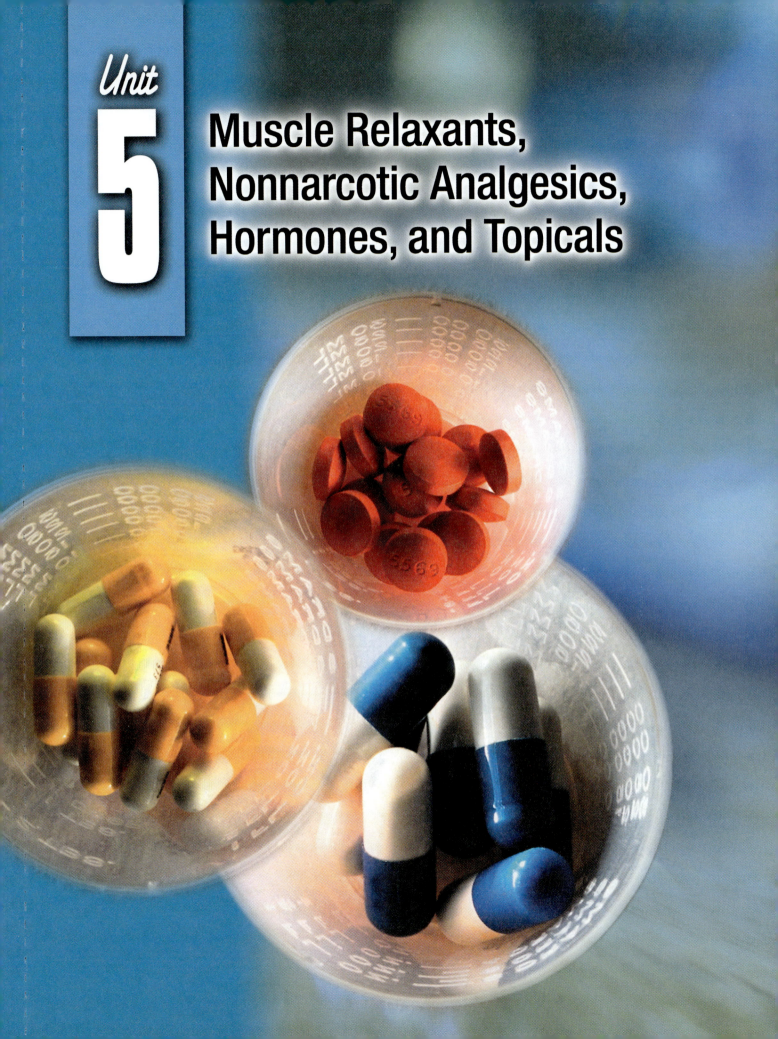

Unit 5
Muscle Relaxants, Nonnarcotic Analgesics, Hormones, and Topicals

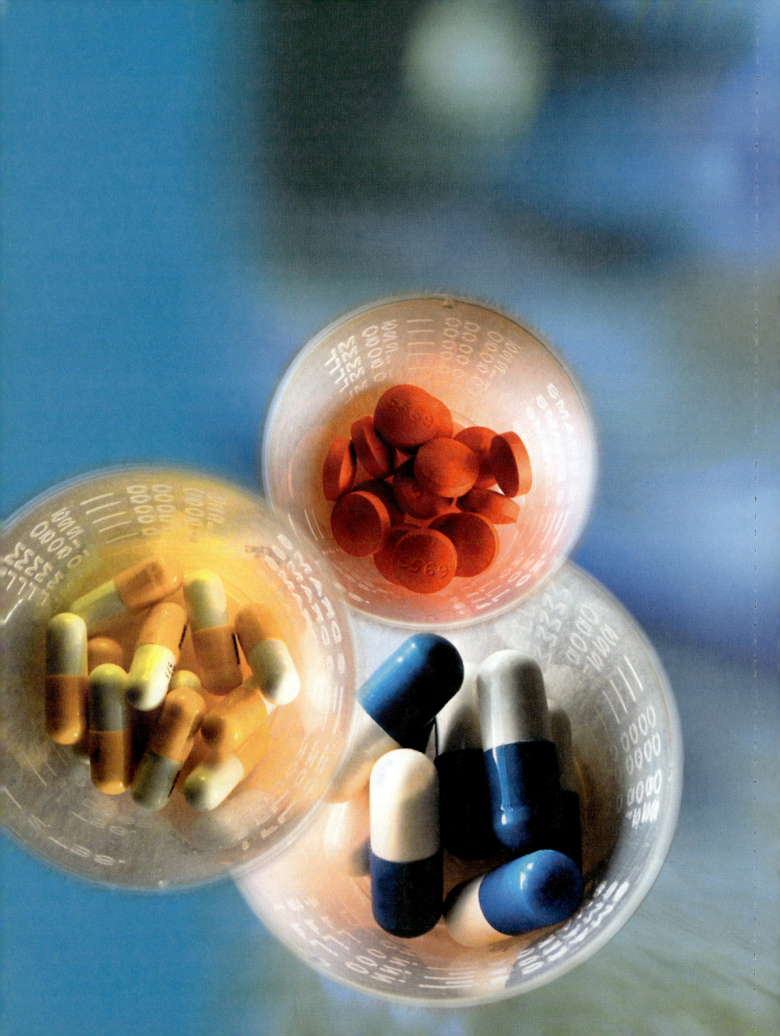

Muscle Relaxants, Nonnarcotic Analgesics, and Anti-Inflammatories

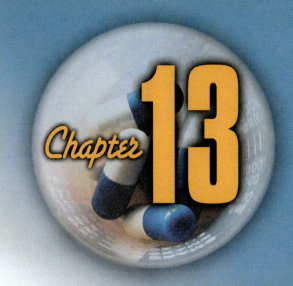

READING DRUG LABELS AND MEDICATION ORDERS

1. You receive the following prescription, and you identify the label shown as the corresponding product available in the pharmacy.

   Rx Mobic 7.5 mg #60 bid

   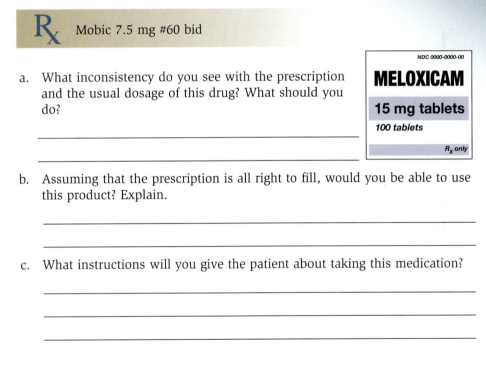

   a. What inconsistency do you see with the prescription and the usual dosage of this drug? What should you do?

   b. Assuming that the prescription is all right to fill, would you be able to use this product? Explain.

   c. What instructions will you give the patient about taking this medication?

2. You receive the following prescription.

   Rx Enbrel 50 mg SC weekly

   a. What class of drug is this?

b. What are the recommended injection sites for this medication, and should they be rotated?

_____
_____
_____

3. You receive the following prescription.

   ℞ Ibuprofen 200 mg I-IV daily prn

   a. As this prescription is written, is it Rx or OTC?

   _____

   b. What is the maximum daily dose of ibuprofen?

   _____

   c. What instructions should you give the patient about taking this medication?

   _____
   _____
   _____

4. You receive the following prescription.

   ℞ Norflex 100 mg ½ tab bid #30

   a. Is this prescription okay to fill? If not, why?

   _____
   _____
   _____

   b. What is the normal intramuscular dose of orphenadrine?

   _____
   _____

UNDERSTANDING THE LARGER MEDICAL CONTEXT

1. Why is it more beneficial to use nonnarcotic analgesics than narcotic analgesics?

2. Define muscle relaxant.

3. What side effect is common among all muscle relaxants?

4. How is osteoarthritis different from rheumatoid arthritis?

5. What role does cyclooxygenase play in pain and inflammation?

6. How do nonsteroidal anti-inflammatory agents work?

7. Why are opiates combined with NSAIDs?

8. What are advantages and disadvantages to using DMARDs?

9. What is gout and how is it treated?

10. What are common side effects of NSAIDs?

COMMUNICATING IN THE PHARMACY

1. A patient comes to your pharmacy to get ibuprofen. What should the patient be told about taking this medication?

2. A doctor calls your pharmacy. She wants to switch one of her patients from a COX-2 inhibitor and needs to know what long-acting NSAIDs are available. How should the pharmacist respond?

3. The same doctor calls your pharmacy and wants to know if Plaquenil can be taken with acetaminophen. What do you tell the doctor?

4. Mr. Johnson is refilling his prescription for colchicine at your pharmacy and tells you that his attacks of gout are getting worse. What can you tell Mr. Johnson about his attacks?

5. A mother comes to your pharmacy to purchase calamine lotion and 81 mg aspirin. She asks if there is anything else that will help her son's chicken pox. What do you do?

___

DISPENSING AND STORING DRUGS

What auxillary labels would you put on the following medications?

1. Skelaxin

2. etodolac

3. celecoxib

4. penicillamine

5. colchicine

6. methocarbamol

7. Norflex

8. Lioresal

9. all NSAIDs

10. etodolac

11. nabumetone

12. celecoxib

13. Ultram

14. cyclophosphamide

15. Rheumatrex

16. Enbrel

What is important about the production and storage of the following solutions?

17. colchicine

18. Enbrel

19. ketorolac

20. cyclophosphamide

21. What ailments are gold compounds used to treat? (Search on MedlinePlus.)

PUTTING SAFETY FIRST

Does the requested dose match the typical medication dose in the following orders? If not, provide the typical dosage for each medication.

1. colchicine 0.6 mg daily
   _____

2. acetaminophen 650 mg q4h
   _____

3. Enbrel 25 mg weekly
   _____

4. infliximab 250 mg IM every 8 weeks
   _____

5. Mobic 7.5 mg daily
   _____

6. Celebrex 50 mg daily
   _____

7. Toradol 10 mg tid for 10 days
   _____

8. EC ASA 625 mg tid
   _____

9. chlorzoxazone cap 250 mg tid
   _____

10. methotrexate 20 mg weekly
    _____

PUZZLING THE TECHNICIAN

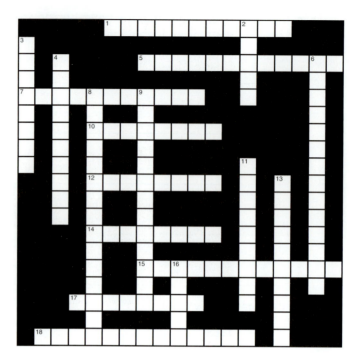

Across

1. prostaglandin analog used to counter the GI side effects of NSAIDs
5. prodrug that is converted to meprobamate
7. type of drugs originally isolated from the bark of the white willow tree
10. brand name for the first COX-2 inhibitor available
12. generic name for Lioresal
14. brand name for allopurinol
15. NSAID used in neonates to prevent some forms of cardiac failure
17. type of pain that originates from the organs
18. can develop in children exposed to viral infections and aspirin therapy

Down

2. deposits of sodium urate around a joint
3. inflammation of the bursa
4. characterized by tinnitus, dizziness, headache, confusion
6. type of arthritis that is degenerative
8. muscle relaxant similar to tricyclic antidepressants
9. neurotransmitter that controls muscle cells
11. brand name for an NSAID/prostaglandin analog
13. type of arthritis that is autoimmune
16. category of drug for slowing the progression of rheumatoid arthritis

PUZZLING TERMINOLOGY

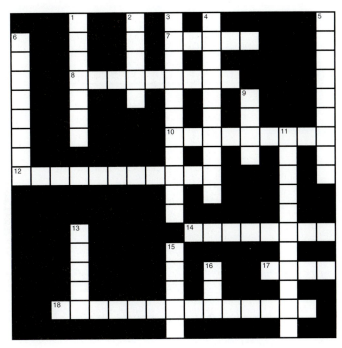

Across

7. an anti-inflammatory, analgesic, and antipyretic drug that is not scheduled; used to treat arthritis and for other indications such as pain and inflammation
8. joint inflammation; persistent pain due to functional problems of the joints
10. agents used specifically to reduce muscle tension
12. a class of nonnarcotic analgesics that have both pain-relieving and antipyretic (fever-reducing) properties
14. sharp, stabbing pain from the organs
17. an enzyme that is present in the synovial fluid of arthritis patients and is associated with the pain and inflammation of arthritis
18. a degenerative joint disease resulting in loss of cartilage, elasticity, and thickness

Down

1. dull, throbbing pain from skin, muscle, and bone
2. deposits of sodium urate around a joint
3. fever-reducing
4. mild salicylate intoxication, characterized by ringing in the ears, dizziness, headache, and mental confusion
5. pain relieving
6. inflammation of a bursa
9. an enzyme that is present in most body tissues and produces protective prostaglandins to regulate physiological processes such as GI mucosal integrity
11. analgesics used for pain, inflammation, and fever that are not controlled substances
13. a syndrome that can develop in children who have been exposed to chicken pox or other viral infections and are given aspirin
15. an agent that can potentially modify the progression of rheumatoid arthritis
16. a neurotransmitter that binds to specific receptors on the membranes of muscle cells, beginning a process that ultimately results in muscle contraction

Hormones

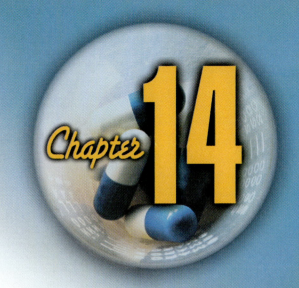

Chapter 14

READING DRUG LABELS AND MEDICATION ORDERS

1. You receive the following prescription, and the drug label shown is the product you pick up from the pharmacy shelf.

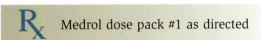
Medrol dose pack #1 as directed

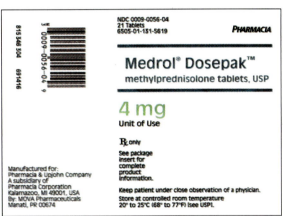
Reproduced with permission of Pfizer Inc. All rights reserved.

a. Does the drug label correspond to the product indicated in the prescription? If not, why?

_____
_____
_____
_____

b. What daily dosing instructions should the patient receive for taking the prescribed medication?

_____
_____
_____
_____
_____

Name _____ Date _____

2. You receive the following prescription, and the drug label shown is the product you pick up from the pharmacy shelf.

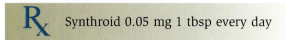
Synthroid 0.05 mg 1 tbsp every day

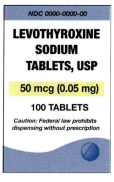

a. Does the drug label correspond to the product indicated in the prescription? If not, why?

_____
_____
_____
_____

b. What dosing instructions should the patient receive for taking the prescribed medication?

_____
_____
_____
_____

3. You receive the following prescription, and the drug label shown is the product you pick up from the pharmacy shelf.

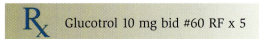
Glucotrol 10 mg bid #60 RF x 5

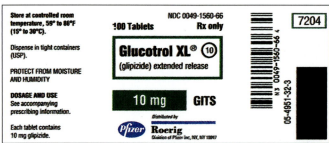
Reproduced with permission of Pfizer Inc. All rights reserved.

a. Does the drug label correspond to the product indicated in the prescription? If not, why?

_____
_____

b. To what drug class does this medication belong and for what medical condition is it typically used? Explain the response the body has to this medication.

_____
_____
_____
_____

c. What side effects are associated with this drug?

_____
_____
_____

4. You receive the following prescription for a 14-year-old patient who weighs exactly 44 kg. The drug label shown below is the product to be dispensed, and you are to dispense the 12 mg cartridge.

> ℞ Humatrope 0.35 mg/kg weekly, given in daily SC INJ

a. What is the total weekly dose? Show your calculation.

_____
_____

b. What would the daily dose be? Show your calculation.

_____
_____

c. If the strength is 4 mg/mL, what will be the daily volume of injection? Show your calculation.

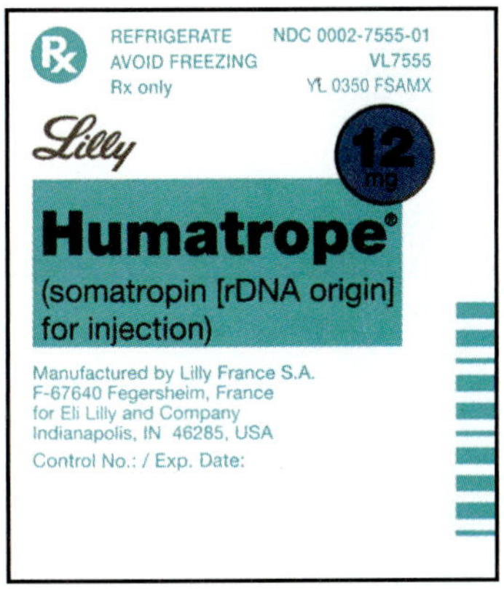

_____
_____

d. How is this product stored?

_____
_____

Humatrope label:
REFRIGERATE NDC 0002-7555-01
AVOID FREEZING VL7555
Rx only YL 0350 FSAMX
Lilly 12 mg
Humatrope®
(somatropin [rDNA origin] for injection)
Manufactured by Lilly France S.A.
F-67640 Fegersheim, France
for Eli Lilly and Company
Indianapolis, IN 46285, USA
Control No.: / Exp. Date:

©Copyright Eli Lilly and Company. All Rights Reserved. Used with Permission. ®HUMATROPE is a registered trademark of Eli Lilly and Company.

UNDERSTANDING THE LARGER MEDICAL CONTEXT

1. Why is it important to exercise caution when using beta blockers in diabetic patients?

_____
_____
_____

2. Name the four types of diabetes and identify the characteristics of each type.

_____
_____
_____
_____
_____
_____

3. What are the signs and symptoms of cretinism, and how is it treated?

4. What are some causes of male impotence that are not related to medication?

5. What happens in the body during menopause, and what are common symptoms experienced by menopausal women?

6. What might cause a potential false-negative and a potential false-positive in a home pregnancy test?

7. What is the difference between an osteoclast and an osteoblast?

8. What role do glucocorticoids and mineralocorticoids play in the body?

9. Why are there no oral insulin preparations?

10. What are signs and symptoms of hyperthyroidism?

COMMUNICATING IN THE PHARMACY

1. What instructions might a patient receive when picking up her first prescription of Fosamax?

   _____
   _____
   _____
   _____

2. A regular patient comes into your pharmacy for a refill of glipizide. You notice she is walking with a distinctive limp, which you have not noticed before. The patient explains that she has developed a blister from her shoe. Why would you bring this to the attention of the pharmacist, and what might the pharmacist say to the patient?

   _____
   _____
   _____
   _____

3. A doctor calls your pharmacy with a question about a patient with hypogonadism. The doctor wants to know what testosterone products are available, and which would be easiest for the patient to administer. What products might the pharmacist recommend?

   _____
   _____
   _____
   _____

4. A 30-year-old female is starting to use oral contraceptives for the first time, and she asks you what side effects she will experience. You direct her to the pharmacist. What do you expect the pharmacist will tell her?

   _____
   _____
   _____
   _____

5. A nurse calls the hospital pharmacy and wants you to discontinue a patient's order for prednisone. You check the profile and notice that the patient has been on 15 mg of prednisone for the last 30 days. What do you tell the nurse?

   _____
   _____
   _____
   _____

DISPENSING AND STORING DRUGS

Where would the following medications be stored in the pharmacy?

1. Fosamax 70 mg

2. teriparatide

3. alprostadil

4. Synthroid

5. zoledronic acid

What auxiliary labels would you put on the following medications?

6. Fosamax 10 mg

7. Ortho Tri-Cyclen

8. AndroGel

9. metronidazole

10. Lantus

11. sildenafil

12. A local doctor calls your pharmacy with questions about bioidentical hormone replacement therapy. In particular, he wants to know which form of estrogen is bioidentical. Use the Web site of the North American Menopause Society (www.menopause.org) to find which form of estrogen he is looking for.

    _____
    _____
    _____
    _____

13. How many menstrual cycles would a woman expect to have if she were using Seasonale?

    _____
    _____

PUTTING SAFETY FIRST

Does the dose match the medication? If not, give a common dose.

1. calcitonin-salmon, 1 spray in each nostril bid

   _____
   _____

2. Protropin 0.3 mg/kg total weekly dose

   _____
   _____

3. Levoxyl 100 mg every day

   _____
   _____

4. Glucotrol XL 10 mg bid

   _____
   _____

5. metformin 850 mg bid

   _____
   _____

6. Humulin R 25 units am, and 12 units pm

   _____
   _____

7. Lantus 10 units am, 15 units pm

   _____
   _____

8. azithromycin 1000 mg x 1 dose

9. acyclovir 200 mg 5 times a day for 5 days

10. oxytocin 10 units postdelivery

PUZZLING THE TECHNICIAN

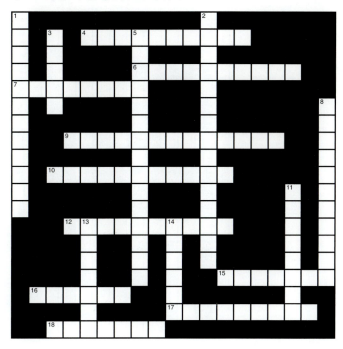

Across

4. brand name for methylergonovine
6. antibiotic of choice to treat gonorrhea
7. longest-acting type of insulin
9. type of exercise that helps maintain bone mass
10. injectable contraceptive given every three months
12. estrogen and nicotine increase the risk of occurrence
15. injectable contraceptive given once a month
16. brand name of teriparatide
17. contraceptive patch
18. where estrogens are produced in the body

Down

1. when blood glucose falls below 70 mg/dL
2. regular recurrence in cycles of 24 hours in the human body
3. genital herpes is this type of infection
5. thyrotoxicosis
8. brand name of the oral contraceptive approved to treat acne
11. brand name of the drug that is a 4:1 combination of T_3 and T_4
13. brand name for vardenafil
14. quickest-onset type of insulin

PUZZLING TERMINOLOGY

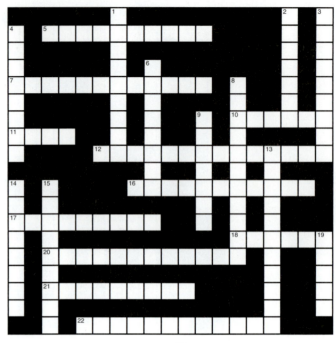

Across

5. pure, synthetic hormones that emulate the effects of progesterone, which prepares the uterus for the reception and development of the fertilized ovum
7. a deficiency of hormone production and secretion
10. a type of diabetes characterized by insulin insufficiency or by the resistance of the target tissues to the insulin produced
11. a neuropeptide secreted by the hypothalamus that stimulates the secretion of growth hormone by the pituitary
12. a deficiency of thyroid activity that results in a decreased metabolic rate, tiredness, and lethargy in adults and causes cretinism in children
16. cells that form bone
17. system composed of glands and other structures that elaborate internal secretions, called hormones, that are released directly into the circulatory system
18. a cell or an organ that is affected by a particular hormone
20. reduction or weakening of bone mass
21. hormones that stimulate the growth of reproductive tissue in females
22. blood glucose less than 70 mg/dL

Down

1. diabetes caused by drugs
2. a sore
3. abnormal hairiness, especially in women
4. a disease caused by overproduction of steroids or by excessive administration of corticosteroids over an extended period
6. a disease characterized by a life-threatening deficiency of glucocorticoids and mineralocorticoids that is treated with the daily administration of corticosteroid
8. cells that resorb bone
9. a gland that produces hormones that stimulate various body tissues to increase their activity level
13. painful intercourse
14. the return of some of the output of a system as input so as to exert some control on the process
15. hormones produced in males in the testes and in females in the ovaries
19. insulin-dependent diabetes, in which the pancreas has no ability to produce insulin

Topicals, Ophthalmics, and Otics

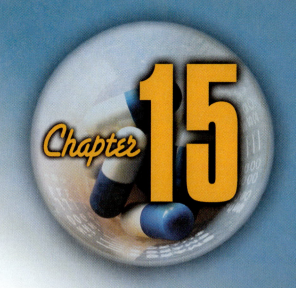

Chapter 15

READING DRUG LABELS AND MEDICATION ORDERS

1. You receive the following prescription.

   Rx tretinoin cream 0.05% apply daily for wrinkles

   a. You identify Retin-A cream 0.05% as the product available. Is this the correct product? If not, then why?

   _____
   _____
   _____

   b. How does this product work?

   _____
   _____
   _____

   c. What should the patient be told about using this product?

   _____
   _____
   _____

2. While you are working in the pharmacy, a doctor calls down and asks you to send up some Bactroban ointment to treat a cultured pressure sore on a patient. You have Bactroban 2% nasal cream in the pharamcay. Would you send up that product. If not, why?

   _____
   _____
   _____
   _____

3. Is something wrong with the following prescription? If so, what is the problem?

> ℞ Johnny Jones, Temovate topical, 0.05%.
> Apply four times a day for one month to diaper area

4. Is something wrong with the following prescription? If so, what is the problem?

> ℞ Auralgan 1 drop in left eye two times daily

5. Is something wrong with the following prescription? If so, what is the problem?

> ℞ TobraDex in left ear twice daily

UNDERSTANDING THE LARGER MEDICAL CONTEXT

1. You receive a prescription for Differin gel.

   a. What problem does the patient have?

   b. The above patient has had reactions to other gels in the past. She wants to ask her doctor for something different. What do you think the pharmacist might recommend?

2. As a technician do you have to worry about the same drug interactions whether the drug is prescribed PO or topically? Explain your answer.

3. Many OTC products are available for ringworm. What are they? Which is the preferred product? What might be the deciding factor when choosing a medication?

4. What is the difference between a cream and an ointment? Can creams and ointments be interchanged? Which is more often prescribed by a dermatologist and why?

5. What is acne?

6. Why can eyedrops be used in the ear, but eardrops cannot be used in the eye?

7. What is the difference between open-angle glaucoma and narrow-angle glaucoma? Which is more common?

8. As a pharmacy technician, what can you do to help patients prevent phototoxicity?

COMMUNICATING IN THE PHARMACY

1. A patient brings in the following prescription and asks you what he needs to know about the medication. What information should be provided to the patient?

   Rx lindane lotion UAD

   _____
   _____
   _____
   _____

2. A patient brings in the following prescription and asks you how to use it. What information should be provided to her?

   Rx Cerumenex UAD may rpt x 1

   _____
   _____
   _____
   _____

3. Mrs. Hollond recently started lisinopril for her hypertension. She was working in her garden and developed sunburn for the first time in her life. She wants your help selecting a sunscreen because she "can't make heads or tails of SPF, UV-A, or UV-B." How will you explain the differences among the notations?

   _____
   _____
   _____
   _____

4. Mr. Holloway is an elderly man who brings in a prescription for erythromycin eye ointment. He has absolutely no idea how to use it. Write out the directions for applying the eye ointment in language the patient will understand.

   _____
   _____
   _____
   _____

5. A doctor calls up your pharmacy. He is very angry because you dispensed an almost empty bottle of Xalatan to one of his favorite patients. What do you tell the doctor?

   _____
   _____
   _____
   _____

6. Mr. Brown has a prescription for two different eyedrops. He applies them four times daily. What must he be told regarding the use of these drops together?

   _____
   _____
   _____

7. Mary Jones has head lice, which her mother says she acquired at day care. Her mother does not have a prescription and wants to get an OTC medication. She is concerned that the OTC medications are not as effective. What will you tell her?

   _____
   _____
   _____

DISPENSING AND STORING DRUGS

Where should the following medications be stored? Indicate an answer for both in the pharmacy and in the patient's home.

1. Xalatan

   _____
   _____

2. dorzolamide

   _____
   _____

3. BenzaClin

   _____
   _____

4. erythromycin opthalmic ointment

   _____
   _____

5. Vigamox

   _____
   _____

What auxiliary labels would you put on the following medications?

6. BenzaClin

7. Retin-A

8. Dovonex

9. Ciprodex

10. Ciloxan

11. Using MedlinePlus, find which eyedrops for glaucoma have the longest-lasting effect.

PUTTING SAFETY FIRST

Does the indication match the drug? If not, list what the drug is commonly used for.

1. pyrethrins for ringworm

2. Botox for wrinkles

3. benzoyl peroxide wash for sunburn

4. tretinoin for wrinkles

5. azelaic acid for acne
   _____

6. Cerumenex for narrow-angle glaucoma
   _____

7. tacrolimus for eczema
   _____

8. imiquimod for ear infections
   _____

9. eflornithine for dandruff
   _____

10. fluorouracil for actinic keratosis
    _____

Name _____ Date _____

PUZZLING THE TECHNICIAN

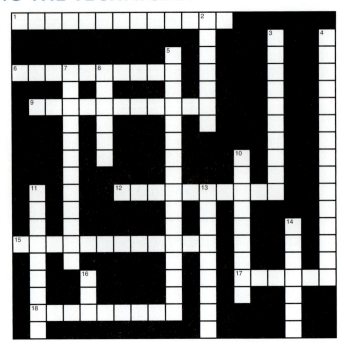

Across

1. generic name for the PO drug used to treat glaucoma
6. inhibits growth of microorganisms, but does not kill them
9. generic name for Trusopt
12. solar lentigines
15. red pustule, common in men after shaving
17. keratococonjunctivitis
18. top layer of the skin

Down

2. brand name of a psoriasis medication that has a maximum dose of 100 g per week
3. OTC drug extracted from chrysanthemums
4. generic name for pHisoHex
5. precancerous condition caused by overexposure to the sun
7. generic name for Sporanox
8. brand name for the drug used to treat xerostomia
10. destroys spores
11. skin condition caused by excessive secretion
13. oxybenzone and para-aminobenzoic acid are components of this
14. tricyclic antidepressant used to treat atopic eczema
16. coal tar

PUZZLING TERMINOLOGY

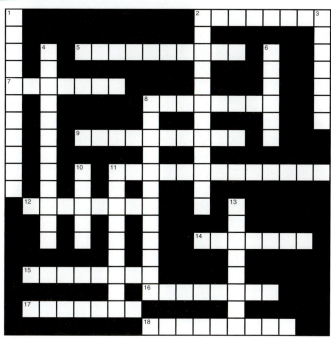

Across

2. a boil; caused by a staphylococcal infection of a sebaceous gland and the associated hair follicle
5. a skin infection characterized by redness and warmth, local pain, edematous plaque with sharply established borders, chills, malaise, and fever; a form of cellulitis
7. this type of dermatitis is an inflammatory reaction produced by contact with an irritating agent
8. sweat glands found in the axillary, perineal, and genital regions
9. coalescent masses of infected hair follicles that are deeper than furuncles
11. an excessive response to solar radiation in the presence of a sensitizing agent
12. itching
14. earache
15. a superficial, highly contagious skin infection; characterized by small red spots that evolve into vesicles, break, become encrusted, and are surrounded by a zone of erythema
16. a fungus that infects the horny (scaly) layer of skin or the nails; also called tinea
17. chronic dermatologic disorder involving inflammation of the skin of the face; also called acne rosacea
18. a skin disorder characterized by patches of red, scaly skin that are slightly raised with defined margins; usually occurs on the elbows and knees but can affect any part of the body

Down

1. an infestation of lice
2. an inflammation of a hair follicle by a minute, red, pustulated nodule without involvement of the surrounding tissue
3. simple tube-shaped sweat glands that are numerous on the palms of the hands and the soles of the feet; regulate body temperature
4. an inflammation of the skin, usually on the face and neck, that is caused by increased activity of the sebaceous glands at puberty
6. a hot, itchy, red, oozing skin inflammation; also called dermatitis
8. the liquid in the front portion of the eye
10. virally caused epidermal tumors
11. minute red spots on the skin due to the escape of a small amount of blood
13. a chronic eye disorder characterized by abnormally high internal eye pressure that destroys the optic nerve and causes partial or complete loss of vision

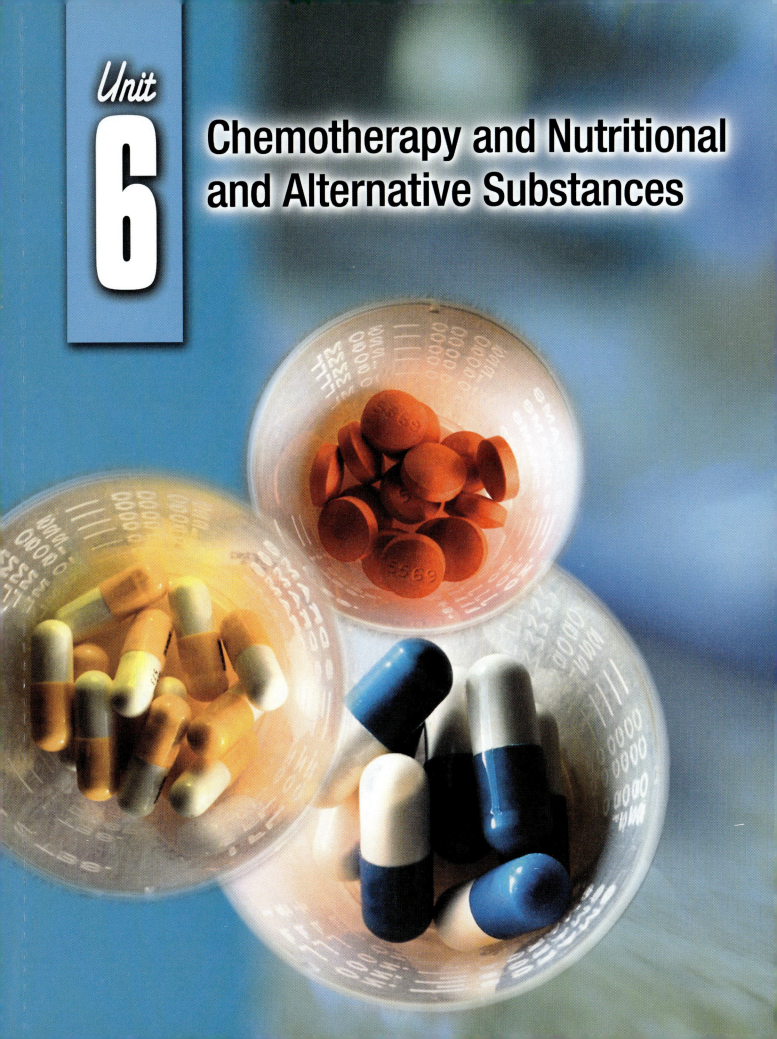

Unit 6
Chemotherapy and Nutritional and Alternative Substances

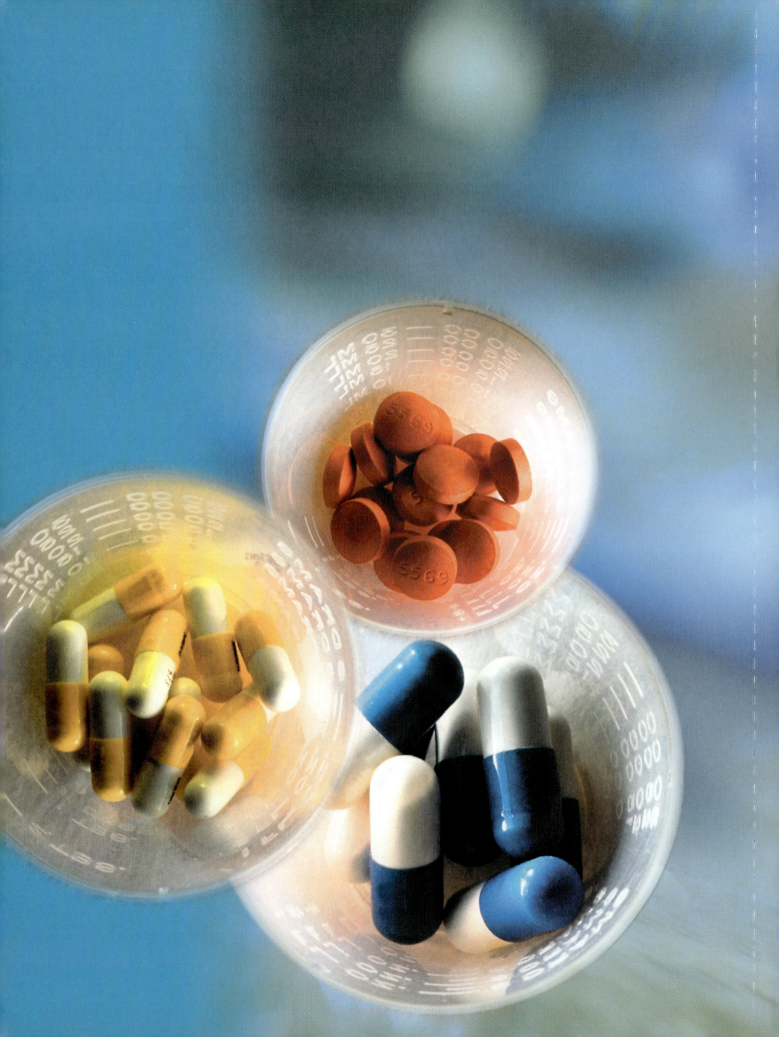

Recombinant Drugs and Chemotherapy

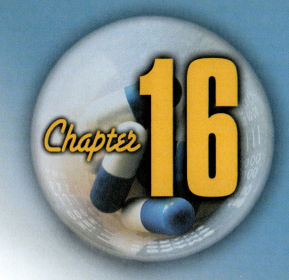

Chapter 16

READING DRUG LABELS AND MEDICATION ORDERS

1. Mr. Kelly is currently being treated for colon cancer. He is 47 years old, 70 inches tall, and weighs 215 lbs. He is starting FOLFOX-6 as his new regimen. The regimen details per cycle are as follows.

    Eloxatin 85 mg/m^2 on day 1

    leucovorin 400 mg/m^2 on day 1

    5-fluorouracil bolus 400 mg/m^2 on day 1

    5-fluorouracil continuous infusion 3000 mg/m^2 over 46 hours on days 1 and 2.

    a. Using the calculator at www.globalrph.com/bsa.cgi, what is this patient's calculated BSA?

    b. If the concentration for the 5-FU is 50 mg/mL, how many milliliters will the bolus be?

    c. Three important facts to know about the FOLFOX regimen is that the oxaliplatin must be given at the same time with the leucovorin, it is not compatible with any sodium chloride-containing solutions, and it is usually in a concentration of 3 mg/mL to 5 mg/mL. Considering these facts, what would be an appropriate diluent and volume for the leucovorin?

    d. How many vials of Eloxatin will be required for three cycles of therapy?

e. The calculated dose for the 5-FU continuous infusion is 6450 mg. If Mr. Kelly is set to receive this medication through an outpatient infusion pump at a rate of 3 mL/hr for the duration of the infusion, how many milliliters must be provided for the course of therapy?

2. Mr. Kelly undergoes three cycles of therapy without improvement. His oncologist decides to add Erbitux to his treatment regimen at a dose of 400 mg/m². The drug label shows the drug to be dispensed.

    a. What is his resulting dose?

    b. How many vials will be required per dose?

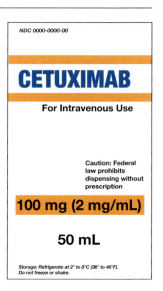

3. Mr. Hamilton has advanced prostate cancer, and he has been given the following prescription. The label indicates the drug to be dispensed.

 Lupron Depot 22.5 mg IM x 1 dose

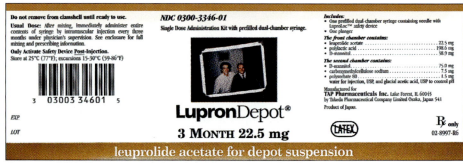

Courtesy of TAP Pharmaceuticals Inc., Lake Forest, IL. Used with permission.

   a. The resultant volume will be 2 mL. Is this volume appropriate for the intramuscular route? If not, why?

   b. When do you expect Mr. Hamilton to come back for another injection?

4. Mrs. Baribeault is currently being treated with ABVD, a regimen with a high incidence of anemia. She has a hemoglobin of 9.6, which is being treated with Epogen with the following instructions.

 Epogen 40,000 units SC once a week

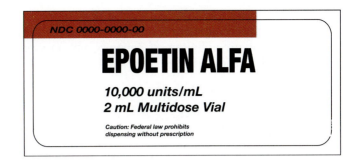

a. How many milliliters will be required per dose?
_____

b. How many vials will be required per dose?
_____

5. Mrs. Prince, a breast cancer survivor, presents the following prescription.

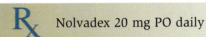 Nolvadex 20 mg PO daily

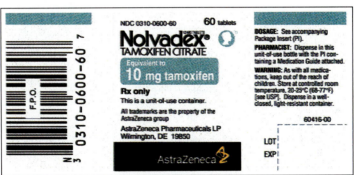

Used with permission of Astrazeneca.

a. How many milligrams will Mrs. Prince receive in a month?
_____
_____

b. How would you write the instructions for the prescription label?
_____
_____

6. Mrs. Anthony, a patient currently in postrenal transplant, is being started on Zenapax. The order follows. How many milliliters of Zenapax will be used for the product shown in the drug label?

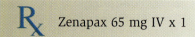
Zenapax 65 mg IV x 1

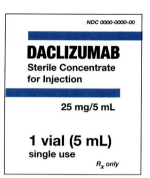

7. Mrs. Brady gives you the following prescription.

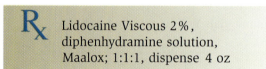
Lidocaine Viscous 2%,
diphenhydramine solution,
Maalox; 1:1:1, dispense 4 oz

   a. How many milliliters of each ingredient will be in the product?

   b. If the patient mistakenly swallows the whole bottle at once, how many milligrams of lidocaine will she receive?

8. Mrs. Blanchard is being treated with carboplatin-paclitaxel for ovarian cancer. Her regimen is as follows. She is 65 inches tall and weighs 160 lbs.

   Paraplatin AUC = 5

   Taxol 175 mg/m^2

   a. Using the calculator at www.globalrph.com/bsa.cgi, what is the patient's BSA?

   b. If the concentration for the Taxol vial is 6 mg/mL, how many milliliters of Taxol will be used per dose?

   c. The pharmacist calculates the Paraplatin dose to be 500 mg. How many milliliters of Paraplatin must be used if the concentration is 10 mg/mL?

UNDERSTANDING THE LARGER MEDICAL CONTEXT

1. Mr. Reynolds is due to receive vincristine 2 mg. The handwriting on the prescription is a bit messy, and you cannot read if the route of administration is IV or IT (intrathecally). What is your opinion of giving vincristine by either of those routes?

2. Mrs. Allen is on epoetin for anemia secondary to chronic renal failure. She has been on 40,000 units weekly. Her current hemoglobin is 12.7, and her hematocrit is 39%. What would you expect to happen to her dose today?

3. A new monoclonal antibody on the market is named Natizumab. Would this be a possible medication for patients with severe allergies to yeast? Why or why not?

4. Mr. James just received a kidney transplant and is starting on full immunosuppressive therapy. What is immunosupression and what are some complications of this condition?

5. The current trend in chemotherapy is to convert to oral therapy whenever possible. For patients on parenteral 5-FU, what may be an option?

6. If you are exposed to an antigen, which cells would provide you with protection from being re-infected eight years from now?

7. What may be an option if a patient is at high risk for cardiotoxicity due to higher cumulative doses of doxorubicin?

8. What medications are useful in treating a type I hypersensitivity reaction?

9. What is the difference between Neupogen and Neulasta?

COMMUNICATING IN THE PHARMACY

1. Mrs. McMillan calls the pharmacy for a refill for her Casodex. Why might you question the pharmacist about that request?

2. Mr. Daniels is finishing his last cycle of cisplatin, which has been implicated in delayed nausea and vomiting. His nurse calls you looking for a pill to keep him from being sick later. What drug do you expect to see in his prescription profile?

3. A nurse calls you and asks you to send some Roferon A for a patient. You see that some Intron A has been checked and is ready to be sent to the floor. Is this an acceptable interchange? If not, why?

4. A physician calls the pharmacy and asks if you have vincristine. What should you ask the physician?

5. Ms. Fitts, a hemophiliac, has been admitted to your hospital for treatment of acute blood loss. What medication should you confirm is in stock at the blood bank?

DISPENSING AND STORING DRUGS

What are the proper auxiliary labels for the following drugs?
1. tacrolimus capsules

2. capecitabine tablets

3. Panretin tablets

4. daunorubicin IV

5. pilocarpine tablets

Where or how should the following drugs be stored?
6. Adriamycin IV vials

7. Faslodex IV

8. Neulasta

9. Xeloda

10. sirolimus liquid

11. megestrol suspension

12. arsenic IV

13. Gleevec capsules

    _____

14. bevacizumab IV

    _____

15. Taxotere IV

    _____

PUTTING SAFETY FIRST

Does the requested dose match the typical medication dose in the following orders? If not, provide the typical dosage for each medication.

1. Xeloda 1 mg PO q8h prn anxiety

   _____

2. filgrastim 6 mg SC x 1

   _____

3. leucovorin 1 mg PO daily

   _____

4. vincristine 20 mg IT x 1

   _____

5. Erbitux 550 mg IV x 1

   _____

6. Kytril 32 mg IV x 1

   _____

7. tamoxifen 200 mg PO daily

   _____

8. Gleevec 500 mg PO daily

   _____

9. Taxol 320 mg IV daily

   _____

10. CellCept 1000 mg PO bid prn rejection symptoms

    _____

Identify the interactions between the following drugs.

11. tamoxifen and Premarin

    _____

12. Prograf and Maalox

    _____

PUZZLING THE TECHNICIAN

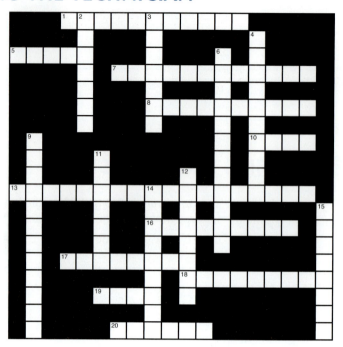

Across

1. cells that digest antigenic cells
5. interferon type produced by T lymphocytes
7. generic for Neoral
8. second-line drug for colorectal cancer
10. site of mucositis and ulceration as complications of anticancer drugs and radiation
13. therapeutic category for Simulect
16. recombinant product for cystic fibrosis
17. drug that prevents cardiomyopathy in patients taking doxorubicin
18. generic for Vepesid
19. Interferon ____ 2a is Roferon A
20. brand name for gefitinib

Down

2. angiogenesis inhibitor
3. two brand names for erythropoietin growth factors are Epogen and this drug
4. only proteasome inhibitor on the market
6. immune process that identifies cells to be phagocytized by macrophages
9. generic name for Temodar
11. tablet for dry mouth
12. hormone antagonist injection given every three months for breast cancer
14. brand name for factor VIII
15. brand name for arsenic trioxide

PUZZLING TERMINOLOGY

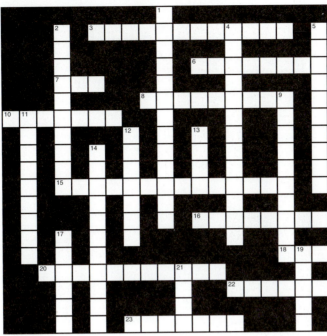

Across

3. labeling antigenic material so that it is more readily identified and destroyed by macrophages
6. small circular rings of DNA that are found in bacteria
7. a single-cell antibody produced in laboratories and used in cancer immunotherapy
8. the condition in which a tumor is inactive with no cell division or growth; typically, a goal of chemotherapy
10. reproducing identical copies of a gene by DNA technology
15. a technique that uses living organisms or parts of organisms for specific purposes
16. the part of plasmid DNA that starts protein production
18. a chemical that stimulates the bone marrow to produce blood cells
20. a replacement plasma protein that is necessary for blood coagulation and is not produced in a hemophilic
22. lymphocytes that respond directly to antigens by producing clones; involved in cellular immunity
23. cancer tumors that are widely distributed and are not localized

Down

1. drugs that prevent the body from rejecting foreign solid organ transplants
2. the portion of plasmid DNA that stops protein production
4. the reading of information from a DNA strand onto an RNA strand, which then serves as a messenger
5. lack of responsiveness of cancer cells to chemotherapy
9. a disorder that occurs when normal cellular control mechanisms become altered; characterized by uncontrolled cellular growth and the development of abnormal cells; also referred to as cancer
11. a network of vessels that carry lymph, the lymph nodes, and the lympoid organs including the tonsils, spleen, and thymus
12. the original site where a cancer tumor develops
13. a single strand of DNA formed in an early step of the recombinant DNA process; serves as a template for the second strand
14. cells that rid the body of antigens, toxins, and cellular debris by ingesting the foreign substance and digesting it
17. antibody-producing lymphocytes that are involved in humoral immunity
19. tumors that form a solid mass and can be palpated
21. an agent that stimulates the bone marrow to produce specific white cells, such as the granulocytes

Vitamins, Nutritional and Alternative Supplements, Antidotes, and Emergencies

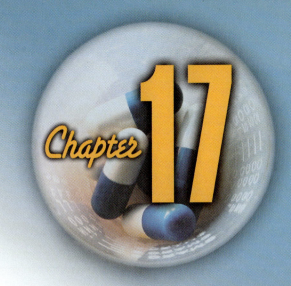

READING DRUG LABELS AND MEDICATION ORDERS

1. You receive the following prescription, and the drug label shown is the product you pick up from the pharmacy shelf.

   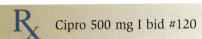
   Cipro 500 mg I bid #120

   a. Is this prescription okay to fill as written? If not, why?

   b. What medical condition does this medication typically treat?

   c. Using the medication indicated in the drug label, how many tablets would you dispense to fill this prescription?

2. You get a new order for a patient while you are working in the emergency room pharmacy. The patient's chart indicates a diagnosis of arsenic poisoning. You find penicillin vk, 150 mg tablets on the pharmacy shelf.

   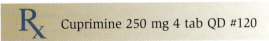
   Cuprimine 250 mg 4 tab QD #120

   a. What is wrong with this prescription as written?

b. Does the drug you found on the pharmacy shelf correspond to the prescribed drug? If not, why?

c. Is this dose correct for the diagnosis? If not, what would the correct dose be?

d. How should the prescribed drug be taken?

3. While working in the emergency room pharmacy, you receive a stat order. The doctor needs an empiric dose for acute digoxin toxicity.

   a. What products are available for treating digoxin overdose?

   b. What is the empiric dose for acute digoxin toxicity?

4. You receive the following prescription at your pharmacy. After searching unsuccessfully for this medication in your drug reference, you notice that the prescription was written by a naturopathic practitioner.

   > **R_x** Prostate Rx (saw palmetto) 1 cap daily

   a. Is this a prescription item? Explain your answer.

   b. What is the daily recommended dose of saw palmetto?

   c. Identify the side effects associated with saw palmetto.

UNDERSTANDING THE LARGER MEDICAL CONTEXT

1. What is the difference between the four different salts of calcium (gluconate, chloride, carbonate, and acetate)?

2. Two types of total parenteral nutrition are available. What are they and what are the differences between them?

3. What regulations exist for nutritional supplements and OTC herbs?

4. What are the steps in the gastric lavage procedure?

5. What are the steps to treat an emergency MI?

6. What are typical causes of water deficit?

7. What are typical symptoms of volume excess?

8. Why is tonicity important when preparing IV fluids?

9. What are the main issues surrounding the use of alternative medicine to treat disease?

10. In case of biologic attack, what role can the pharmacy technician play?

COMMUNICATING IN THE PHARMACY

1. A patient comes into your pharmacy looking for a calcium supplement. She is examining a bottle of calcium carbonate and a bottle of calcium gluconate. She asks you which one is better. What should she be told?

2. A nurse calls the pharmacy and wants to know if there are special precautions for adding regular insulin to a patient's TPN. What information should she receive?

3. At your pharmacy, you notice that as a patient is paying for a refill of his prescription for fluoxetine, he is also purchasing a bottle of St. John's wort. Is there a reason to alert the pharmacist? If so, why?

4. A patient comes into your pharmacy looking for echinacea. She wants to know if there are any problems taking it with her "real" drugs. What do you think the pharmacist will tell her about this drug?

5. The emergency room doctor calls the pharmacy and tells you that the Mucomyst oral solution in the Blue Alert cart has turned purple. He wants the solution replaced stat. What do you tell the doctor about Mucomyst?

DISPENSING AND STORING DRUGS

Are the following medications available over the counter or by prescription?
1. calcium acetate

2. vit B_{12} 1000 mcg INJ

3. dong quai

4. activated charcoal

5. vitamin K

6. penicillamine

7. pyridoxine 2 mg

8. vitamin D₂

9. calcium gluconate

10. Jevity Plus

11. Find, list, and compare the amount of B vitamins in the nutritional products Jevity 1 cal and Ultracal per 8 oz serving.

PUTTING SAFETY FIRST

Does the dose match the medication? If not, give a common dose.

1. Mucomyst for acetaminophen toxicity 140 mg/kg PO

2. riboflavin 500 mg bid

3. calcium acetate 750 mg daily

4. melatonin 10 mg hs

5. St. John's wort 300 mg tid

6. When mixing TPN, which elements have to be separated so as not to precipitate in the bag?

7. What is the purpose of epinephrine in a CODE emergency kit?

8. What are signs and symptoms of inhaled anthrax infection?

_____
_____
_____
_____

9. What are the signs and symptoms of ricin poisoning?

_____
_____
_____
_____

10. Many people take individual vitamins in excessive quantities with the theory of more is better and healthier. Explain why it is important to limit the amount of over-the-counter fat-soluble vitamins (A, D, E, K).

_____
_____
_____
_____
_____
_____
_____

PUZZLING THE TECHNICIAN

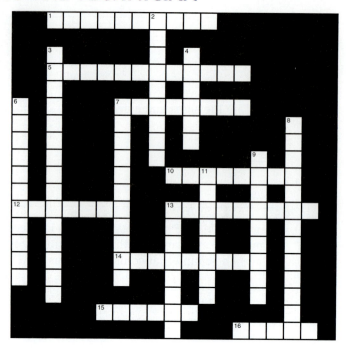

Across

1. type of overdose penicillamine is used to treat
5. chemical name of vitamin C
7. virus that has been mostly eradicated throughout the world, but still exists in laboratories
10. brand name for the drug used to treat acetaminophen overdose
12. class of drugs that can cause respiratory depression in high doses
13. hormone produced by the body that produces drowsiness
14. brand name of flumazenil
15. cation that promotes fluid retention in the body
16. drugs metabolized by this organ are affected by ingestion of grapefruit

Down

2. herb used to shorten the duration of the common cold
3. vitamin B_5
4. herb used for hyperlipidemia
6. paired with glucosamine, this substance is believed to prevent enzymes from destroying cartilage
7. Nature's Prozac
8. first step to eliminate poison
9. solution with a lower concentration of particles than the body fluid contains
11. calcium salt that is the quickest to get into the bloodstream
13. protein-calorie malnutrition that results in growth retardation

PUZZLING TERMINOLOGY

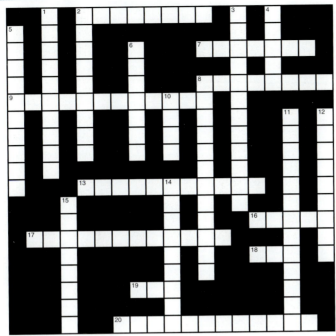

Across

2. a blood pH below 7.35; a metabolic condition due to excessive loss of bicarbonate or sodium
7. by way of, or pertaining to, the intestine
8. a type of protein-calorie malnutrition that results in growth retardation
9. demineralization and weakening of the skeleton, caused by a deficiency of vitamin D in adults
13. alcohols having the properties of vitamin E
16. a toxin derived from the castor bean that acts by inhibiting protein synthesis
17. a neurotoxin that blocks the release of acetylcholine at the neuromuscular junction, resulting in muscular paralysis
18. an amino acid-dextrose-lipid formulation used for parenteral nutrition; often called three-in-one
19. feeding a patient through the veins
20. substances that dissociate into ions in solution and are thus capable of conducting electricity

Down

1. a solution with a higher concentration of particles than body fluids contain
2. a blood pH above 7.45; a metabolic condition due to excessive loss of potassium or chloride
3. vitamins that are excreted in the urine and are not stored in the body; vitamin C and the B vitamins
4. plants or plant parts extracted and valued for their savory, aromatic, or medicinal qualities
5. therapy for poisoning that consists of establishing the airway and providing cardiopulmonary resuscitation (CPR); maintaining body temperature, nutritional status, and fluid and electrolyte balance; and preventing circulatory collapse, hypoglycemia, uremia, and liver failure
6. a time-saving process used when preparing a three-in-one TPN, in which all electrolytes except phosphate are put into a small-volume parenteral bag and then transferred into each batch
8. any disorder of nutrition
10. a system to communicate that a patient is in a life-threatening situation
11. a procedure to wash out or irrigate the patient's stomach
12. a material used in treatment of poisoning by animal venom
14. a solution with a lower concentration of particles than body fluids contain
15. organic substances that occur in many foods and are necessary for the normal metabolic functioning of the body